# EMDR AS YOU ARE

## 12 Experts on Moving from Protocol to Presence

Edited by

ROTEM BRAYER, MED, LPC

# Advance Praise

"EMDR as You Are* is the book the EMDR community needs. My friend and colleague Rotem Brayer has long taken a 'keep it real' approach to EMDR and clinical work. His commitment to amplifying the voices of real EMDR therapists and making EMDR therapy more accessible to the people they serve is admirable. I highly recommend this anthology to novice and seasoned EMDR therapists alike."

— Jamie Marich, PhD

Author of *EMDR Made Simple*, *Dissociation Made Simple*, and *Trauma and the 12 Steps*

Founder of The Institute for Creative Mindfulness

"Like a gathering of wise colleagues from an EMDR resource team, *EMDR as You Are* reveals how each contributor has adapted and evolved their practice, offering unique perspectives shaped by their own conceptual, personal, and clinical frameworks. The result is a rich tapestry of insight that celebrates the synergistic potential of EMDR when practiced with openness, courage, creativity, authenticity, and a genuine curiosity to explore what might be possible."

— Jocelyn Rose

Senior accredited MBACP

Coauthor of *Psychedelic-Assisted EMDR Therapy*

"*EMDR as You Are* is a must-read for EMDR-trained professionals at all levels. The different perspectives offered through various lenses will make this book a unique and welcome addition to your library."

— Agnes Wohl, LCSW

Certified EMDR therapist

Diplomate of the American Academy of Experts in Traumatic Stress

"Reading *EMDR as You Are* felt like looking into a mirror and seeing an EMDR therapist facing self-doubt and uncertainty. It's empowering to learn that even EMDR's most respected figures have walked similar paths. Their candid journeys and diverse influences offer deep comfort and inspiration. It's like holding the distilled wisdom of many EMDR books in one powerful, accessible volume."

— Alemayehu Tibebe, MA, MPH

EMDR therapist and basic consultant in positive and transcultural psychotherapy

"This collection is exactly the kind of resource I wish I'd had after completing EMDR basic training. Each therapist's voice offers a unique and authentic perspective, which reminds us that EMDR is not a one-size-fits-all modality. The honesty, practical wisdom, and real-world applications encourage therapists to trust the foundational principles of EMDR while staying true to themselves. *EMDR as You Are* is a wonderful resource for both new and seasoned EMDR clinicians."

— Aly Webster, LCPC

Creator of *EMDR Cognition Cards*

"This book beautifully illustrates that EMDR, while grounded in a strong foundation, is a nuanced, messy, and beautiful healing practice that allows for clinical intuition and the integration of different modalities. *EMDR as You Are* counters the rigid lens through which many of us were trained, encouraging therapists to trust themselves and their unique approaches."

— Tiffany Simmons, LPC, LAC

EMDRIA-approved consultant

"*EMDR as You Are* should be required reading for EMDR clinicians. Each chapter offers something distinct, so there is something for everyone. The diversity of voices and experiences is beautiful, yet it all stays deeply faithful to Francine Shapiro's original vision for EMDR."

— Debra "Deb" Sprague, MEd, LPC

EMDRIA-approved consultant

"*EMDR As You Are* brings together a wealth of highly skilled EMDR providers who generously share their knowledge on topics ranging from well-loved books to the role of attachment in EMDR work. With its eclectic approach, readers will discover creative, research-informed resources they can integrate into their clinical work with clients."

— Crystal Horning, LPC, PLLC
EMDRIA-approved consultant

"Rotem Brayer is brilliant in his ability to build community and strong, life-giving support through his book. The format welcomes us as it also generously and wholeheartedly gives the very reflections we most want from our mentors. There is a deep sense of being part of a global and passionate group of therapists who are changing the world, starting with authentic connection to their own deep work and inviting us to do the same."

— Julie H. Richards, MS, LPCC
Developmental and relational trauma therapist

"Rotem Brayer's *EMDR as You Are* is a valuable contribution to our community. Both new and seasoned EMDR therapists can benefit from the perspectives and toolboxes of the many experienced clinicians in this book. Because it showcases a range of approaches within the EMDR framework, therapists can discover their own therapeutic style and increase the likelihood of remaining engaged with the model. *EMDR as You Are* reinvigorated my passion for healing through EMDR."

— Jenny Jacoben, LPC
EMDR-certified therapist

"Many clinicians struggle with using EMDR consistently and confidently in day-to-day practice. EMDR as You Are addresses the most common questions therapists have, offering grounded guidance that helps you move through fear and uncertainty. Highly recommended for all EMDR clinicians!"

—Kyle Poon, MEd
EMDRIA-approved trainer
Creator of Calm with Kyle

Library of Congress Cataloging-in-Publication Data available.

ISBN: 979-8-9948060-0-5

Ebook ISBN: 979-8-9948060-1-2

Library of Congress Control Number: 2026915243

Publisher: Insight Psychotherapy, LLC

# About the Editor

Rotem Brayer, MEd, LPC, is a licensed professional counselor, certified EMDR therapist, EMDR consultant, and EMDR educator. He is the founder of The EMDR Learning Community
(emdr-learning.com), a global community that brings EMDR clinicians together for training, consultation, and practical tools for integrating EMDR with other evidence-based approaches. Based in Denver, Colorado, Rotem is in private practice and spends his time consulting on cases, coaching EMDR therapists, and supporting clients as they heal from trauma and attachment wounds; he is also the author of *The Art and Science of EMDR: Helping Clinicians Bridge the Path from Protocol to Practice.* and the editor of *EMDR As You Are: 12 Experts on Moving from Protocol to Presence.*

# Contents

# Acknowledgments

This book has been on my mind for more than two years. It took time to shape the idea, find the right contributors, and bring all of the pieces together into the book you are about to read. Along the way, I leaned on more people than I can properly capture in a few lines, but there are a few I want to name here.

Ari and Noam, my kids, thank you for filling my life with joy. Getting to watch you grow, seeing your curiosity in action, and getting to know who you are becoming is the greatest privilege of my life.

To the contributors of this book: Thank you for trusting me with your stories and your clinical wisdom. You made time, you leaned in with vulnerability, and you brought real heart to these chapters. This book exists because of your generosity.

Marisa Solis, thank you for your rare mix of precision and care. You went above and beyond as my editor and book coach, and you helped me keep going when it got hard. This book is better thanks to you.

To the members of The EMDR Learning Community: Thank you for the way you show up, share honestly, and keep learning out loud. Your questions, reflections, and willingness to exchange ideas have shaped this book more than you know. We've built something that feels like family, and I'm grateful to be part of it.

With gratitude,

Rotem

# Introduction

Most EMDR therapists leave basic training feeling both inspired and unprepared. In the training room, the steps make sense, the scripts are clear, and the possibilities seem endless. Then you sit down with a real client, and the work gets less predictable.

The manual on your desk is consistent and structured, but the human in front of you is not.

Questions come quickly: *Where do I start? How do I keep my client safe? What if I get stuck?* When you're new to EMDR, these moments can make the therapy feel more complex than the training suggested. Some therapists hesitate, and some stop using EMDR altogether. They believe in it, but they don't feel confident enough yet to trust themselves.

*EMDR as You Are* is here to bridge the gap between basic training and real-session confidence. It offers personal stories, professional strategies, and hard-won wisdom from 12 expert EMDR therapists who have stood where you are now. They've faced uncertainty, learned through trial and error, and found ways to adapt EMDR to the person in front of them while still staying grounded in the standard protocol. Their diverse journeys reveal that mastery comes through practice, humility, and authenticity.

EMDR is structured yet deeply individualized. As a therapist, you master the principles and the eight phases. Then you learn to use them like a second language. The steps stop feeling like something you're reciting and start feeling like something you can rely on when the session doesn't go the way you expected. From there, you tailor the work to the client.

No two EMDR sessions are ever the same, and they shouldn't be. In this work, knowledge counts, but attunement counts more. Your presence, your responsiveness, and your ability to meet your client where they are can be the difference between a session that feels mechanical and one that truly moves.

## How I Got Here

Several years ago, I stood in the same place EMDR therapists just out of basic training find themselves in: holding a manual full of steps that made sense on paper but feeling suddenly dubious about how to use them in real life. After a tough session, I remember thinking, *Is this really working, or did I buy into the hype?* I was tired, unsure, and, if I'm honest, a little desperate for something solid to hold on to.

What helped wasn't a perfect script. It was people. A small circle of colleagues who wanted to share what was working, be honest about what wasn't, and help each other stay in the work long enough to get good at it. We celebrated each other's wins, talked through stuck places, and kept returning to the basics when things felt messy. Over time, that circle grew into The EMDR Learning Community.

Since then, I've used EMDR successfully with clients facing trauma, depression, anxiety, attachment wounds, addictions, and physical symptoms that hadn't shifted with other approaches. I've also used EMDR with people who don't meet criteria for any diagnosis but feel stuck in patterns they're ready to change. Those experiences, along with ongoing learning from consultation and community, fuel my passion to share this book with you. Listening to colleagues changed my EMDR practice. It gave me more confidence in the room and helped my clients move, even when the work was complex. My hope is you'll find that same kind of support and clarity in the words of the highly experienced EMDR clinicians in this book.

Basic training is the beginning; competence grows through practice, feedback, and time. Training gives you structure; the therapy room asks you to use EMDR in the living, unpredictable space between two nervous systems.

## How This Book Is Different

EMDR literature is increasingly crowded with new protocols and procedures, and the amount of material can be overwhelming. So why add another book to the shelf? Because *EMDR as You Are* is different in tone and purpose. It combines clear clinical thinking with real-session decision-making, shared with unusual transparency by highly experienced EMDR clinicians. In their own words, they offer practical interventions you can use right away, along with honest accounts of what it took to build confidence and skill over time.

This book complements basic training, ongoing consultation, and ethical decision-making. It is not a substitute for EMDR therapy training or consultation. It's designed to be helpful for all trained EMDR therapists, whether you're early in your journey or an experienced clinician looking for renewed confidence and clarity.

*EMDR as You Are* features a dozen EMDR therapists speaking candidly about various aspects of their work, such as:

- how they explain EMDR to clients
- what they do when a client gets stuck
- what influences shaped their approach
- which interventions have become their go-to tools

Each contributor answered questions of their choosing from a shared list and wrote out their responses in their own words. You'll get a clear sense of each therapist's unique style. You'll see common patterns emerge across chapters, as well as differences of opinion. You'll see the human side of expertise too: even highly respected EMDR therapists have had doubts, made mistakes, and questioned whether they were doing it "right."

Over time, they had powerful breakthroughs, made crucial adaptations, and found a way to practice EMDR that fits who they are. They share how a range of integrations—including IFS, ego state work, attachment-focused approaches, ecotherapy, and Jungian concepts—is possible while keeping the standard EMDR protocol close and adapting to the person in front of them. Many offer step-by-step guidance you can use right away for common client challenges, including when processing gets stuck, dissociative responses show up, or attachment wounds shape what happens between you and your client.

As you read, choose one idea from each chapter to test, either in a session, a role-play, or a consultation. Notice what shifts when you apply it, and bring your questions back to your consultation space.

## EMDR as You Are, and as You Become

To be the best EMDR therapist you can be, you have to bring yourself fully into the work. Not the polished, idealized version you imagined in training, but the real you, with instincts, quirks, and influences shaped by your history and your teachers. Despite what some voices might imply, you don't have to change who you are to become a good EMDR therapist. You learn the protocol deeply, and then you let it meet your authentic presence. That's often what helps clients feel safe enough to explore the most raw, unguarded aspects of their experience—the places that are unseen, unspoken, and still unhealed.

This book is meant to remind you that your voice, your way of tracking the room, and your way of being with people matter. The protocol and the adaptive information processing (AIP) model are your foundation. They come alive when they meet your humanity. When you bring your full self into the room, you make it safer for your clients to do the same. That is where real healing happens.

If you find yourself at that intersection—wanting to believe in EMDR but uncertain how to use it with confidence—I invite you into the worlds of our contributors. Together, they show something more generous than "one right way." They show a living practice that honors both structure and individuality.

I hope this book gives you clarity, flexibility, and a wider range of options when sessions become complex.

Enjoy the journey,

Rotem

# Chapter 1

# Fidelity Meets Creativity: Jackie Flynn

Jackie Flynn, EdS, LMHC-S, RPT-S, is an EMDRIA-approved EMDR trainer, consultant, registered play therapist supervisor, and author of *EMDR with Kids Flip Chart: A Play-Based Tool for Trauma Processing, Nervous System Regulation, and the Transformation of Adaptive Behaviors* and *Little Gecko's Broken Tail: A Book to Introduce EMDR Therapy to Children*. She helps children and families heal from trauma using creative, developmentally attuned, neuroscience-informed methods.

Jackie is also the founder of EMDR Playground, a supportive community for EMDR-trained therapists who work with children and adolescents. Her approach integrates EMDR therapy with play therapy, sandtray therapy, and other expressive modalities to foster regulation and adaptive processing. She also creates practical resources that make complex ideas engaging for therapists and children.

Jackie's work reflects deep respect for the developing nervous system and the essential role of play in trauma healing. Through training, consultation, and creative tools, she helps therapists maintain EMDR fidelity while adapting to the unique needs of children. Jackie's teaching stands out for its clarity, accessibility, and clinical expertise, rooted in her belief in the healing process.

## Which books have influenced your work as a therapist?

***Being a Brain-Wise Therapist: A Practical Guide to Interpersonal Neurobiology* by Bonnie Badenoch**

This book shifted my view of the therapeutic relationship, showing therapy as an embodied, co-regulatory process, not just interventions. Badenoch offers practical ways that neuroscience informs clinical work. I learned the value of therapist self-regulation and attunement, especially with traumatized children, from this book. Now, I prioritize presence and relationship over technique in all EMDR phases, especially with young clients.

***Man's Search for Meaning* by Viktor E. Frankl**

Frankl's writing changed my approach to trauma work by emphasizing the importance of meaning-making in the healing process. Frankl's experiences illustrated that finding purpose, even in the midst of suffering, is central to resilience. I now honor each client's search for meaning, especially in EMDR's installation phase. Frankl's insights deepen my work by inspiring me to center clients' evolving self-stories and emphasize transformation, rather than simply symptom relief.

***Eye Movement Desensitization and Reprocessing (EMDR) Therapy: Basic Principles, Protocols, and Procedures* by Francine Shapiro**

This foundational text provides ongoing guidance in my EMDR practice and training. Shapiro's emphasis on adhering to the standard protocol while adapting for complex cases anchors my work. Her explanation of the adaptive information processing (AIP) model continues to shape my case conceptualization. I frequently turn to this book because it reinforces the idea that EMDR is about supporting the brain's innate healing capacity—a core concept I apply to both my clinical work and teaching.

## How do you explain EMDR to your clients?

I prioritize clear, simple explanations of EMDR that are tailored to each client. My primary focus is to make the process feel natural and accessible. This helps clients understand EMDR by connecting it to something intuitive and avoiding overwhelming details. I usually introduce it this way:

*EMDR therapy helps your brain do what it was built to do—process and make sense of experiences. Just like your body digests food, your mind digests life. When something overwhelming or traumatic happens, that process can get interrupted, and the memory gets stored in a raw, unprocessed way. EMDR helps the memory move again—not to erase it, but to help it land in the past where it belongs.*

*The EMDR process is based on the adaptive information processing model. This model suggests that your brain naturally wants to heal; it just needs the right conditions to facilitate this process. EMDR activates a stuck memory and uses bilateral stimulation—such as eye movements, tapping, or sounds—to help your brain reprocess it. As that happens, emotional intensity begins to settle, new insights may arise, and the memory integrates more adaptively. The EMDR process shifts from something that hijacks your nervous system to something that feels resolved.*

*EMDR follows a structured eight-phase protocol designed to keep the process safe and supportive. You are aware of the entire process and remain in control of your own actions. My job is to guide, not direct; your system leads the way.*

> *Just like your body digests food, your mind digests life.*

I've found that this language helps clients feel grounded. They need a map, not a lecture. They respond really well to something that helps them understand their feelings, promises the possibility of healing, and explains that EMDR supports what's already within them.

## What advice do you have for new EMDR therapists?

**Know that EMDR is not just a tool or technique—it's a comprehensive therapy model.** This is one of the most important things a newly trained EMDR therapist should understand. Each of the eight phases—history taking, preparation, assessment, desensitization, installation, body scan, closure, and reevaluation—has its own purpose, supporting healing from start to finish. When we treat EMDR as something applied only during reprocessing, we miss the depth and intention of the approach. EMDR is not just about bilateral stimulation; it concerns how trauma is stored, how the nervous system holds experience, and how healing unfolds with enough support and structure.

**Know that fidelity matters—especially if you want to be creative.** You need to be grounded in the model to adapt to it. That is what allows you to bring in approaches such as parts work, sandtray, or movement without slipping into something that only vaguely resembles EMDR. The phases are there for a reason. When we are anchored in them, we can be flexible in ways that are still safe, still effective, and still doing the work. I've learned that the more creative I become, the more tightly I need to hold on to the framework. That's what gives the work its strength.

**Remember that phases 1 and 2 aren't boxes to check.** I continually revisit phase 1, history taking, staying curious about new targets, noticing emerging material, and pivoting as needed. I listen for unmet needs, unresolved patterns, and subtle signs of secondary gains that might slow progress. Phase 2, preparation, is where we introduce safety, resourcing, and nervous system support. These elements are rarely one and done; I revisit them often. Some clients return to resourcing during reprocessing, while others need it to be integrated into every session. Returning to resourcing isn't backtracking; it's fidelity to the nervous system.

*Returning to resourcing isn't backtracking;*
*it's fidelity to the nervous system.*

**Slow down in phase 8.** Reevaluation is another area where many EMDR therapists move through too quickly. This phase is not just about knowing what to target next. It's also a chance to support deeper integration. I use this time to track changes in how the client navigates the world. Are they responding differently? Are they reclaiming parts of themselves? Are they using resources more naturally? Phase 8 invites us to reflect, integrate, and stay connected to the ongoing arc of healing, not just plan for the next target.

**Learn to attune to clients.** Doing this changed everything for me. I used to focus on what clients said, but now I notice signals my body sends. Our nervous systems connect in subtle ways, often where the most important information lies. You don't need to know what it means every time. Just notice and stay curious. That alone can create safety through connection.

**Don't do this alone.** Early on, I presented imperfect sessions during the consultation. I asked awkward questions. I shared sessions I was not proud of, but I kept showing up. That is how I learned—not by getting it perfect, but by staying engaged. EMDR is a layered, complex, and beautiful process. You don't have to know everything; you just have to stay connected to the model, stay curious, and keep showing up. That is more than enough to start.

## What training has had the greatest impact on your practice?

Providing EMDR Through Sandtray Therapy, with Marshall Lyles, in March 2024, transformed my EMDR practice, especially with children and teens. This training demonstrated how sandtray therapy supports every phase of EMDR by honoring metaphor, pacing, and nervous system safety. It emphasized that healing stories often emerge through image and movement, not just words.

Before this training, I already valued creative approaches in my work, but sandtray therapy provided me with structure and language for what I had been sensing intuitively. It encouraged me to trust client pacing and support integration in relational and embodied ways.

A few days later, I attended Marshall's second training, Sandtray, Poetry, and EMDR Processing in the Treatment of Attachment Wounds with Adults. This training added even more depth. It opened up new ways to use expressive tools, such as poetry and metaphor, when working with adult clients. It reminded me that expressive arts are not only for children. Adults often carry attachment wounds that are difficult to access through language. The training showed me how to gently invite those parts of the story forward using image, rhythm, and symbol.

> *Expressive arts are not only for children.*

Both trainings gave me tools and helped me reimagine EMDR therapy across the lifespan. I now integrate sandtray, poetry, and symbolic play with ease, meeting clients where they are and building trust in the healing process.

## What did you intuitively know without formal training?

One thing I intuitively knew how to do in my EMDR practice, even before it was named in a training, was to move and attune with my clients. To share breath, rhythm, and space in a way that felt less like a therapist and a client and more like co-regulators, both present with something sacred.

When bilateral stimulation began, I didn't just sit still and observe; I was actively engaged. I noticed myself breathing in sync with my clients, subtly mirroring the pace of their inhales and exhales while letting the rhythm of my own body provide steadiness. If their foot was tapping or their fingers were moving, I sometimes found my own body moving too—not to imitate but to join. I noticed that when I allowed this subtle resonance, something softened in the room. The client felt less alone. There was a felt sense of connection. We weren't rushing through steps; we were weaving something.

> *When I allowed this subtle resonance, something softened in the room.*

I also found myself offering bilateral stimulation in ways that felt organic to the moment. Sometimes we walked together. Sometimes we used sound or simple shared movement. The protocol remained intact, but the delivery was deeply relational and embodied. I followed the fidelity of the phases but trusted my body to guide the pace.

What I now understand is that this kind of embodied attunement supports the body's social engagement system. It helps the client stay within their window of presence, where trauma can be held and shifted without overwhelm. At the time, I didn't have language for any of that. I just knew the healing happened most deeply when we were in rhythm together.

## What is one therapeutic approach that integrates really well with EMDR?

One integrative approach that fits seamlessly with EMDR is sandtray therapy. It doesn't sit alongside the protocol as an add-on; it becomes the space where the phases of EMDR deepen and come alive. The symbolic and sensory nature of the sandtray allows access to what is stored implicitly—beyond language and linear memory—while still working within the eight-phase model. It offers containment, expression, and flexibility, especially for clients whose nervous systems need a slower, more right-hemisphere approach to trauma processing.

> *The sandtray allows access to what is stored implicitly—beyond language and linear memory—while still working within the eight-phase model.*

I worked with a mother who came to therapy after a miscarriage. Kaia could talk about what happened, but the impact of the loss hadn't fully integrated. Her system was still carrying it tenderly, protectively, but also in distress.

In phase 1, history taking, we gathered background information not only through conversation but also by watching what emerged in the tray. Kaia's first scenes evoked a sense of frozen time, deep quiet, and distance. Without needing to narrate every detail, she was already identifying memory networks that held unprocessed pain. We stayed in phase 1 longer than usual—not out of avoidance, but because her system kept offering more.

Phase 2, preparation, wasn't a single session. It was woven throughout the work. Kaia built resources symbolically by placing a mother-bear figure near a shelter and adding natural elements such as water and fire. These choices weren't random; they reflected how her system found support. Resourcing occurred throughout the process. We explored whether healing would mean forgetting. Grief often showed up as a thread she feared letting go of. The tray provided a form for these tensions, offering space for regulation, support, and insight.

Her target emerged through a sandtray image: the moment she saw the ultrasound with no heartbeat. Kaia's negative belief was "It's my fault." What she wanted to believe was "I did everything I could."

In phase 3, assessment, we explored the worst part and its associated cognition, distress level, and body sensations. In phase 4, desensitization, we processed the memory with bilateral stimulation while Kaia adjusted the scene in the tray as things began to feel different. This was the adaptive shift taking place. Figures were moved and new symbols introduced. Her nervous system began to integrate what had been fragmented.

By phase 5, installation, the positive belief "I did the best I could" began to truly fit. Then we moved to phase 6, body scan. Something still remained, revealed through physical sensations. Kaia placed a small flower beside a stone and said quietly, "She's still with me, just differently now." The body scan reflected that. There was a felt sense of calm, not a disappearance of grief, but a softening.

Phase 7, closure, was about completion with respect. We returned often to earlier resources and used her own images to support regulation between sessions. In another tray, Kaia used the sand for grounding as we breathed together, then took a walk to choose an object of every color of the rainbow. She went home lighter.

In phase 8, reevaluation, we revisited not only the target memory but also the integration of her story. We explored what still needed attention and noticed how she was relating to herself differently. Phase 8 wasn't about closure; it was about continuation with greater capacity and coherence.

When we integrate sandtray therapy with EMDR, fidelity is essential. It lets us work creatively without losing direction. Creativity without structure can drift. But when we stay anchored in the eight phases, we gain the freedom to follow the client's system with care, depth, and precision. This kind of integration deepens right-hemisphere access, offers safety in symbolic form, and enables us to reach pain that transcends words.

## Which EMDR intervention have you found particularly effective?

One therapeutic approach I created and now teach—along with sandtray therapy trainers Alisha Denham and Catherine Denham—is ReWilding EMDR. This integrative method weaves natural elements into each phase of the EMDR protocol while maintaining fidelity. This approach grew out of observing how trauma often disconnects people from their bodies, their environment, and the present moment. Nature, when incorporated into therapy, serves as both a co-regulator and a grounding force. ReWilding EMDR helps clients reengage their senses, access implicit memory, and integrate experiences by restoring connection to the body, relationships, and environment.

> *ReWilding EMDR helps clients reengage their senses, access implicit memory, and integrate experiences by restoring connection to the body, relationships, and environment.*

In phase 1, history taking, we often begin outdoors or use nature-based metaphors. Alongside the AIP model, we explore the client's sensory relationship with the natural world. Some clients identify trauma not only in memory but in their disconnection from safe, natural spaces. A timeline might be built with leaves, stones, or sticks, offering symbolic access to implicit memory and intergenerational patterns.

In phase 2, preparation, we develop regulation through simple practices such as orienting to surroundings, barefoot grounding, or naming natural resources. Clients may choose a tree for stability, water for flow, or fire for resilience. These are not symbolic overlays but embodied, co-regulated experiences. I may guide a brief somatic warm-up outdoors, rotating attention through the body while listening to the sounds of birdsong or the wind. Nature-based poetry, stories, and drawing also help reinforce resources we can return to throughout the phases.

In phase 3, assessment, targets often emerge through creative expression. A client might arrange stones to represent a traumatic moment or sketch a landscape where a memory lives. Negative and positive cognitions emerge through this process, and body sensations often become more distinct and pronounced. Validity of cognition (VOC) and subjective units of disturbance (SUD) ratings are taken in safe outdoor spaces or through imagery of previously created resource settings.

In phase 4, desensitization, I use natural bilateral stimulation, which may include walking side by side on a trail, listening to alternating ocean waves, or tapping thighs while tracking birds in flight. The rhythm of the earth supports regulation and release. Symbolic items, such as stones, may be adjusted as the memory shifts.

In phase 5, installation, the client strengthens the positive cognition through interaction with a natural element. If their new belief is "I am connected," they might anchor it by placing a hand on a tree or breathing in sunlight. These actions reinforce the embodied shift and extend the change beyond the session.

In phase 6, body scan, nature remains a co-regulator. The client may sit on the earth or engage with scent, texture, or sound while moving attention between internal sensations and the external environment. This helps the nervous system settle and integrate.

In phase 7, closure, we mark the end of the session with simple rituals inspired by the four elements, such as creating a wind prayer, stacking stones with intention, or placing feet in a stream. These acts support containment and transition.

In phase 8, reevaluation, we revisit the work through a nature-based mindfulness approach. Clients may return to a resource location and notice how the target feels in body and mind. Shifts in breath, posture, or inner narrative often highlight the depth of integration.

ReWilding EMDR does not complicate EMDR; it reconnects us to something ancient and wise—the body's memory of safety in nature. Fidelity to the eight phases provides structure while allowing creativity. Nature becomes a therapeutic partner, helping clients access the layers of experience that words alone cannot reach.

> *Nature becomes a therapeutic partner, helping clients access the layers of experience that words alone cannot reach.*

## What EMDR success story caught you by surprise?

One EMDR success story that caught me by surprise began with a client on the edge of burnout. Raul was stuck in a job where he was consistently undermined, micromanaged, and at times openly harassed. He came to therapy uncertain about whether to leave. The job was misaligned in every way, yet Raul couldn't imagine stepping away from it. Something in him kept whispering, "Maybe it's me." He felt so stuck that suicidal thoughts had started to creep in—quiet but persistent.

As we explored Raul's history, a long pattern began to emerge. He had often stayed in environments where he felt undervalued. In childhood, caregivers praised his achievements but rarely showed him emotional support. Raul had internalized the belief that he had to prove himself over and over again, and even then, it might not be enough. That core belief—"I am not good enough"—had been shaping his adult life in powerful, limiting ways.

We spent time building resources. One of the most powerful resources came through imagery. Raul imagined standing on a mountainside, solid and steady, feeling the wind and the weight of his own presence. It became an anchor, something he could return to in sessions and in life.

The memory we targeted was a moment when a supervisor publicly criticized him for something he hadn't done. Raul remembered sitting there, taking it, even though it was profoundly unfair. The belief was clear: "I am not good enough." What he wanted to believe instead was: "I am skilled and valuable."

As we moved through bilateral stimulation, Raul's posture began to shift. Initially, there was a profound sense of shame and despair. Soon, he began to sit up straighter. He imagined himself calmly stating the truth, then walking out of that meeting and into the sunlight. That memory no longer had power over him. It wasn't just about what had happened; it was about his ability to respond.

When we installed the new belief, it finally felt true. Raul's voice conveyed confidence. He looked up instead of down. "I am skilled and valuable" wasn't just a phrase—it felt true.

> *"I am skilled and valuable" wasn't just a phrase—it felt true.*

In the days and weeks after that session, things began to move. Raul started asking bigger questions: "Has this job ever aligned with who I am? Have I ever really been seen there? What do I actually want?" The new belief generalized in ways I had not anticipated. He not only left that job but started his own company. The same qualities that once made him vulnerable to exploitation—his attention to detail, his drive to do things well, his deep sense of responsibility—became Raul's strengths.

During a later session, I asked how he was feeling in his body. He paused, then said, "I feel lighter—like I'm not dragging something behind me anymore." There was a new spaciousness in him. Raul didn't need to prove anything. He could just be.

We honored this shift with a small ritual. He chose a stone to keep on his desk as a reminder of what he had reclaimed. That act of closure marked something sacred—not just an end but a return to himself. And in the sessions that followed, it was clear: The belief had taken root, the trauma had integrated, and Raul was no longer stuck in a loop.

What surprised me most was how the very thing that held him back—his relentless need to be enough—became the source of his power. EMDR didn't turn him into someone else. It helped him come home to who he truly was.

## Have you experienced imposter syndrome?

There was a time early in my EMDR journey when I struggled to keep all eight phases organized in my head. I understood the essence of the work, but the structure felt overwhelming due to all the details. So I did what I always do when something matters: I immersed myself. I read and reread Francine Shapiro's book. I memorized the EMDR definition as outlined by EMDRIA. Eventually, I created my own quick reference guide, a phase-by-phase map that helped me stay grounded while still allowing room for the intuitive, relational way I work.

Sometimes what makes an EMDR session feel challenging is remembering all the complexities—what is supposed to happen when. I remember considering this as I sat with a client whose trauma felt layered and diffuse. We weren't moving forward, but we weren't fully stuck either. It was murky. That murkiness helped me recognize that I had lost my bearings in the phases. Now I make it a point to know where I am in any given moment.

In phase 1, history taking, I asked myself whether I had truly assessed readiness for EMDR. *Had I identified clear targets for reprocessing? Had I explored the client's strengths and possible secondary gains or blocks that might be holding us back?*

Phase 2, preparation, invited me to slow down and reconnect. I reviewed how I had explained EMDR and whether the client felt safe enough in the relationship to manage their affect. I made sure our regulation strategies were robust and that the client knew what to expect.

Phase 3, assessment, required me to return to the right- and left-brain integration that the protocol offers. *What image represented the worst part? What negative belief was tied to that image? What would they rather believe? How true did that belief feel? What were the emotions and body sensations that came up?*

Phase 4, desensitization, reminded me to pair the image with the negative belief and stay attuned to pacing. Using bilateral stimulation, I carefully tracked the SUD levels. I stayed close to the process, without pushing, trusting the shifts to emerge in their own time. If the SUD score moved to zero or felt ecologically valid, I knew it was time to move forward.

Phase 5, installation, involved checking in on the positive cognition we had chosen in phase 3, then allowing space for the new belief to strengthen. I helped the client confirm that the belief still fit and paired it with the target memory. We used faster-paced bilateral stimulation to install it so that it would stick.

Phase 6, body scan, brought our attention back to the body. We returned to the target and the positive belief, noticing what showed up somatically. I think of a body scan as a polygraph test exposing any residual material. Any distress was met with more bilateral stimulation to allow further resolution.

> *"I think of a body scan as a polygraph test exposing any residual material."*

Phase 7, closure, reminded me of the importance of regulation. Even—especially—if the target wasn't complete, we used grounding, imagery, and resourcing to help the client leave feeling safe and contained.

Phase 8, reevaluation, returned us to the work with fresh eyes. At the next session, I checked whether the target still held distress and reassessed the belief. If needed, we circled back. If not, we identified the next steps in the broader treatment plan to deepen the work.

What I learned from that session was that structure doesn't stifle intuition; it protects it. Having the eight phases clearly in mind gave me the clarity I needed to move forward. That's why I created my EMDR quick reference guide: to remind myself that fidelity and flexibility are not opposites; they are companions in this work.

> *"Structure doesn't stifle intuition; it protects it."*

## References

Badenoch, B. (2008). Being a brain-wise therapist: A practical guide to interpersonal neurobiology. W. W. Norton & Company.

Flynn, J. (2023). Little gecko's broken tail: A book to introduce EMDR therapy to children. Independently published.

Flynn, J. (2024). EMDR with kids flip chart: A play-based tool for trauma processing, nervous system regulation, and the transformation of adaptive behaviors. PESI Publishing.

Frankl, V. E. (2006). Man's search for meaning. Beacon Press.

Shapiro, F. (2017). Eye movement desensitization and reprocessing (EMDR) therapy: Basic principles, protocols, and procedures (3rd ed.). Guilford Press.

# Chapter 2

# Never Stop Learning: Robin Shapiro

Robin Shapiro, LICSW, MSW, has always found meaning in supporting others. After years of volunteering at crisis clinics and answering calls at the Seattle Counseling Service, serving sexual minorities, she earned her degree from the University of Washington School of Social Work.

Her first job was directing a day treatment program at Seattle Counseling Service, where colleagues joked, "To be in Robin's group, you have to be queer, and you have to be crazy." When federal funding cuts shut down the program, she transitioned to full-time private practice.

Robin has worked as a therapist since 1981 and started practicing EMDR in 1993, the year she married. She enjoys teaching and consulting, and finds profound meaning in empowering people to help others. Her EMDR specialties include working with all levels of dissociation, integrating EMDR with ego state and somatic therapies, and supporting survivors of sexual abuse to heal and, if they wish, create fulfilling sexual lives. In consultation, she helps consultees build their own support and healing. She encourages strong self-care, including making time for fun.

## Which books have influenced your work as a therapist?

***EMDR Toolbox: Theory and Treatment of Complex PTSD and Dissociation*** **by Jim Knipe**

Jim Knipe's wonderfully clear book explores shame, ego states, and other essential concepts for working effectively with a diverse range of challenging clients.

***Complex Integration of Multiple Brain Systems* by Beatriz Sheldon and Albert Sheldon**

This book is a comprehensive compilation of their work on Complex Integration of Multiple Brain Systems (CIMBS), which explores attachment, cognition, and various other factors that support effective therapy. I took six years of classes from them, and the book summarizes it well.

***Treating Trauma-Related Dissociation: A Practical, Integrative Approach* by Kathy Steele, Suzette Boon, and Onno van der Hart**

This book is a comprehensive and insightful exploration of complex trauma. It's one of the most helpful resources I've encountered. It begins with the therapeutic relationship, followed by assessment and treatment planning, and then proceeds through various treatment methods, including EMDR. A must-read!

## How do you explain EMDR to your clients?

I tell clients: *When we experience trauma, our nervous system and brain encode it in a way that keeps us on alert to protect us. This encoding often includes fear, flashbacks, intrusive thoughts, and avoidance of anything that might be a reminder.*

*EMDR gently pressures the memory networks to reduce or eliminate the trauma response. This helps remove bad dreams, intrusive thoughts, nightmares, and flashbacks.*

*When applied gradually, EMDR can reinforce positive feelings and constructive beliefs. It often helps clients connect to their wisest, most grounded state.*

*For EMDR to be effective, clients must first be anchored in a safe, present-moment state. They then link this calm state with the distressing memory so it can be resolved.*

I'll say: *If you don't want to revisit difficult memories, we can use the Four Blinks Version of Flash. You'll focus on a favorite thing or listen to your favorite music while visualizing the old memory locked in a box, and we'll do some blinks.*

Or I'll say: *If you feel ready to face a big memory, we can use the newer EMDR 2.0 approach. This approach puts more pressure on the memory networks by having you do several things at once, which can help clear it from both the brain and the body.*

## What advice do you have for new EMDR therapists?

**Tailor the treatment to each client.** EMDR is a powerful therapy, but you can't consistently deliver it exactly as you were trained. Every client is unique, and you need to tailor the treatment to fit their individual brain, nervous system, and experiences.

> *Every client is unique, and you need to tailor the treatment to fit their individual brain, nervous system, and experiences.*

**Help clients strengthen their sense of the safe present moment.** Have them tap into a memory of when they felt good, or the safety of your office, or the current moment. Ask, "How old were you when that bad stuff happened? How tall were you? How old are you now? How tall? If that abuser tried to attack you now, 30 years later, what could you do to protect yourself? Feel that strength and ability, and tap that in."

**Decide if EMDR is needed right away.** Sometimes you won't do EMDR immediately. If your client has a stable past and only one recent trauma, you may proceed more quickly. Otherwise, take a thorough history to uncover earlier traumas and any lack of secure attachment, safety, or stability.

**Assess your clients' level of dissociation.** Complex trauma, including chronically unsafe or neglectful childhoods, can contribute to personality disorders. Earlier and more severe trauma can train the nervous system to flood the body with endogenous opiates, which create dissociation (not "disassociation," which is incorrect). Dissociation can range from shutting down or spacing out to dissociative identity disorder (DID), where "parts" take turns managing life without awareness of one another. If you're working with clients in this range, consider seeking additional training and extensive consultation.

**Educate yourself.** Read Rebecca Kase's *Polyvagal-Informed EMDR: A Neuro-Informed Approach to Healing*, the second edition of Jim Knipe's *EMDR Toolbox*, Carol Forgash and Margaret Copeley's *Healing the Heart of Trauma and Dissociation with EMDR and Ego State Therapy*, and both of my *EMDR Solutions* books to start. Then take every relevant class or training you can, attend EMDRIA conferences, and read widely about the issues you encounter in your office. Above all, make sure you have a skilled consultant who understands the work, supports you fully, and is flexible rather than rigid.

## What is one therapeutic approach that integrates really well with EMDR?

Ego state therapy is indispensable for EMDR therapists. PTSD displays dissociation, and most clients exhibit complexities beyond simple PTSD. Therapists must assess, clarify, and treat dissociation using both EMDR and ego state therapy.

*Ego state therapy is indispensable for EMDR therapists.*

Ego state therapy differentiates, labels, and heals the neural networks shaped by recurring actions, feelings, or thoughts that influence identity and behavior. For those with early trauma, endogenous opiates may numb intense emotion, prompting new neural networks—the "parts." In DID, parts have specific names, roles, and emotions. Some remain entirely isolated from others.

Ego state work connects the most adult self to all parts and heals the parts that need care. In simple trauma cases, the adult part is guided back in time to bring the younger, traumatized self into the safe present time and place. This is repeated until the younger self fully realizes it's now, it's over, and they are safe with the adult in charge.

For individuals with personality disorders, a strong adult may help younger parts relinquish their roles and allow the adult to take the lead. The adult can revisit earlier moments, giving the younger parts the love and care (April Steele's *Developing a Secure Self*) or forgiveness (Jim Knipe's *EMDR Toolbox*) they needed. This heals the client's most vulnerable parts, allowing the adult to respond to love and distress from a healed, mature perspective.

Ego state therapy is crucial for treating DID. You must identify all parts, establish the adult as the leader, heal the trauma in younger parts, and integrate them into a healthy, present-focused adult. Applying EMDR to the trauma itself can take years, as using it too early can cause further dissociation, intense flashbacks, and loss of the adult self. EMDR might be used earlier with individual parts, but only if they are well contained and strongly connected to the adult.

## Which EMDR intervention have you found particularly effective?

I've found that EMDR for chronic pain, tinnitus (ringing in the ears), long COVID, and multiple chemical sensitivities are particularly effective.

### Chronic Pain

There are at least two ways our bodies experience pain. One is physiological. If you fall down and hurt yourself, the pain signal travels from your body through your nerves to your brain, prompting you to say, "Ouch!" The second way is neurological. This happens when, even after the body heals from an injury, the nervous system may continue to send pain signals to the brain.

> *Even after the body heals from an injury, the nervous system may continue to send pain signals to the brain.*

Neurological pain has been treated many times with EMDR. Mark Grant developed one of the first pain protocols. His work targets the initial injury, subsequent pain, and current pain. In many cases, the pain subsides. I've adapted his protocol by adding imagery and polyvagal calming techniques for even greater effect.

Here's how I apply EMDR for chronic pain.

**Intake**

- When did the pain (or injury, illness, etc.) start?
- How bad is it now?
- When does it hurt the most?
- How has it affected your life?
- What feelings do you have about it now?

**EMDR**

- Use the standard protocol with eye movements, tapping, or other bilateral stimulation (BLS).
- Target the initial injury.
- Target when the pain is most distressing.
- Target losses caused by the pain.
- Target the current level of pain—where it is located—and feelings about it in the present moment.

**Polyvagal calming**

- *Silencing the alarm*: Place your right hand over your left eye. Then, with the same hand, brush firmly behind the left ear, down the neck to the shoulder, then to the elbow, and off the back of the left hand. Switch sides and repeat. Perform 10 times on each side.
- *Negative breathing*: Breathe out fully and completely. Breathe in halfway. Repeat at least 10 times.
- *Grounding*: Feel gravity holding you to your chair, with your feet on the floor. Drop your shoulders. Relax. Look around and notice that you're safe here.
- Explore additional vagal exercises on YouTube at Calm with Kyle.

**Visualizations with slow BLS**

- Find the dial or lever that turns off the pain.
- Imagine pulling the pain out of your body.
- Practice polyvagal exercises and visualizations at home if symptoms return.

## Multiple Chemical Sensitivity

Multiple chemical sensitivity (MCS) occurs when the immune system overreacts to chemicals, scents, or foods that are not actually harming the body. It can be debilitating, causing symptoms such as hives, choking, itching, or other distressing reactions. A colleague once asked if I thought EMDR could help. I suggested that the pain protocol might be effective—and it was. Within 45 minutes, the client's severe symptoms were gone. She was able to leave her house again, wear her favorite perfumes and creams, and eat all the foods she had previously reacted to.

**Intake**

- When did you have the first significant reaction and what triggered it? (Could be as early as birth or as recent as last week.)
- What was your first reaction?
- What do you react to now? What kinds of reactions occur?
- How has this changed or reorganized your life?
- What do you avoid?
- What activities or places do you grieve not being able to enjoy?

**EMDR**

- Apply the standard protocol with eye movements, tapping, or other bilateral stimulation.
- Target the initial reaction and subsequent negative reactions.
- Target distress over the changed life.
- Target current reactions.

**Polyvagal calming**

- *Silencing the alarm*: Place your right hand over your left eye. Then, with the same hand, brush firmly behind the left ear, down the neck to the shoulder, then to the elbow, and off the back of the left hand. Switch sides and repeat. Perform 10 times on each side.
- *Negative breathing*: Exhale completely—empty your lungs fully. Inhale halfway. Repeat at least 10 times.
- *Grounding*: Feel gravity holding you to your chair, with your feet on the floor.

Drop your shoulders. Relax. Look around and notice that you're safe here.

- Explore additional vagal exercises on YouTube at Calm with Kyle.

**Visualizations with slow BLS**

- Identify the dial for the immune responses needed to combat COVID, E. coli, colds, flu, and other infections. Keep that turned on.
- Find the dial or lever for neurologically based reactions. Turn it completely off and lock it down.
- Continue polyvagal exercises and visualizations at home if symptoms reappear.

## Tinnitus

I've treated approximately 30 cases of tinnitus, with most resolving completely. For some clients, the tones return during periods of anxiety but disappear again after polyvagal calming exercises. One client, whose ear ringing sound was rated 8 out of 10 and had worked in construction for 40 years, experienced a reduction to a 4 and was delighted with the improvement. Many others experienced full relief in one to three sessions.

**Intake**

- When did it start? Was there an event or a head injury?
- Is it the same in both ears?
- How loud is it on a scale of 1 to 10? What kind of noise is in the left ear? The right ear?
- What makes the sound change? (Anxiety, outside noises, etc.)
- When is it the most irritating? (Often at night, disturbing sleep)

**EMDR**

- Apply the standard protocol with eye movements, tapping, or other bilateral stimulation.
- Target when it first started, along with any associated event.

- Target when it has been the most distressing.
- Target losses due to tinnitus.
- Say, "Just focus on the sound in that ear [or those ears]. What do you notice in your body right now? What emotion goes with that? How big is it?" Continue processing as long as it keeps changing.

**Polyvagal calming**

- *Silencing the alarm*: Place your right hand over your left eye. Then, with the same hand, brush firmly behind the left ear, down the neck to the shoulder, then to the elbow, and off the back of the left hand. Switch hands and repeat. Perform 10 times on each side.
- *Negative breathing*: Breathe out fully and completely. Breathe in halfway. Repeat at least 10 times.
- *Grounding*: Feel gravity holding you to your chair, with your feet on the floor. Drop your shoulders. Relax. Look around and notice that you're safe here.
- Explore additional vagal exercises on YouTube at Calm with Kyle.

**Visualizations with slow BLS**

- Imagine pulling or pouring the noise out of your ears.
- Find the dial or lever that sets the sound and turn it completely off.
- Practice polyvagal exercises and visualizations at home whenever the sound returns, especially during times of anxiety.

## Long COVID

COVID is real. Long COVID is the nervous system acting as if the infection is still active. I've worked with nine people with chronic long COVID, using the same protocols as for chronic pain, MCS, and tinnitus. We cleared the symptoms out of each of them in one session, never to return.

**Intake**

- When did you get sick?
- What were the worst parts of it?
- What are your current symptoms? How bad?
- Are they constant (usually so) or on and off? (If so, what triggers them?)
- How are you feeling about it right now?

**EMDR**

- Apply the standard protocol with eye movements, tapping, or other bilateral stimulation.
- Target the worst part of the initial illness.
- Target when it's been most distressing.
- Target losses due to illness.
- Notice the current symptom (fatigue, coughing, etc.). What do you notice in your body in response to it? Name the feeling and rate its intensity.
- Continue processing until it improves.

**Polyvagal calming**

- *Silencing the alarm*: Place your right hand over your left eye. Then, with the same hand, brush firmly behind the left ear, down the neck to the shoulder, then to the elbow, and off the back of the left hand. Switch hands and repeat. Perform 10 times on each side.
- *Negative breathing*: Exhale completely—empty your lungs fully. Inhale halfway. Repeat at least 10 times.
- *Grounding*: Feel gravity holding you to your chair, with your feet on the floor. Drop your shoulders. Relax. Look around and notice that you're safe here.
- Explore additional vagal exercises on YouTube at Calm with Kyle.

**Visualizations with slow BLS**

- Find the dial or lever that turns off the symptoms.
- Imagine pulling the symptoms out of your body.
- Continue polyvagal exercises and visualizations at home if symptoms reappear.

## What role does attachment theory play in your EMDR practice?

I was practicing attachment-oriented therapy long before I learned EMDR. Unless clients had perfect lives and only one recent trauma, such as a car accident, I made sure they felt connected, supported, and safe with me before beginning any EMDR work.

I have been practicing EMDR for nearly 32 years. About 10 years ago, I completed the CIMBS training with Albert and Beatriz Sheldon, learning new techniques for fostering connection and initiating processing through the therapeutic bond. I often sit close to clients and say, "You and I are here to be with every thought, every sensation, and every emotion. What are you noticing right now?" Their answer is often fear or shame. Then I offer, "Let me help you hold that."

*Their answer is often fear or shame. Then I offer, "Let me help you hold that."*

As more material surfaces and we reach the first time they experienced that feeling, often in childhood, I bring in EMDR: "So you're thinking about your mother turning away from you, and feeling shame in your gut? How big is that feeling, 0 to 10? Let's go with that." Then add BLS.

I also tell clients with attachment wounds, especially those who may feel abandoned at the end of a session, that they can take my caring home with them: "Where do you feel my caring in your body and brain? When you're missing me, reconnect with that feeling. You get to keep it forever. No extra charge."

I frequently use April Steele's Imaginal Nurturing and Adventuring Spirit protocols (available at www.april-steele.ca) with clients who had poorly attached parents. In Imaginal Nurturing, the adult client returns to the day of birth to hold, adore, accept, and nurture the baby self. In Adventuring Spirit, the adult connects with the two-year-old self, lets the child choose a toy to play with while staying connected, and then invites the child back a few times—building object constancy. This helps clients internalize the sense that you can go away and still be there, loving and available. It's beautiful work.

## What creative modifications have you made to EMDR to address specific populations or presenting issues?

I created the two-hand interweave. This technique involves separating ideas, feelings, or choices physically by holding one in each hand. For example:

- "Hold what you like about that guy in one hand, and what you can't stand in the other. Hold them together—that's the guy you're with."
- "Hold the shame that the kid part of you carries in one hand, and your adult awareness that you are and always were a good human who deserved love in the other. Let the adult hand hold the kid hand, and let that kid know he was always lovable—he just had parents who didn't have the capacity to show him that."
- "Hold your current job in one hand, and the one you're considering in the other. Spend time with that one, then this one. How does that one feel? How about this one?"

If I'm working with a client with OCD I might say: "In one hand, hold how likely it is that everybody at that party will be thinking of you [or how likely it is that you'll be in a car crash, plane crash, etc.]. In the other, rate how scared you are that the thing will happen on a scale of 0 to 10. Feel that fear in your body. Go with that."

Then I process with EMDR. When the fear clears, I return for future template work: "Next time that fear comes up, tell it to be quiet and remind yourself that the chances of that thing happening are 1 in 1,000. Then calm your body down with deep breaths and grounding."

## What self-care practices do you engage in regularly?

I limit my caseload to no more than three DID clients at a time. I also limit my work to no more than 25 face-to-face client hours per week, not including training time. I always make sure to belong to a consultation group. I continue to learn new ways to help clients. Recently, this has included EMDR 2.0, Four Blinks Version of Flash, and some somatic techniques.

I engage in daily aerobic exercise, typically a two- to three-mile walk that takes me through a beautifully wooded park in my neighborhood, along with about 20 minutes of stretching. I also have great friends and make time to see them regularly. I have a loving husband who cooks for me and makes me laugh. I enjoy playing with my silly cat, Lulu. I maintain a gratitude practice, writing at least three things each day for which I feel grateful.

These practices support my work by keeping me present, mindful, and happy. They sustain me personally, which in turn sustains my clinical work; they give me examples I can confidently recommend to clients.

## References

Calm with Kyle. Home [YouTube channel]. https://www.youtube.com/@CalmwithKyle

Forgash, C., & Copeley, M. (Eds.). (2007). Healing the heart of trauma and dissociation with EMDR and ego state therapy. Springer Publishing Company.

Grant, M. (2023). Pain control with EMDR: Treatment manual (8th rev. ed.). Trauma and Pain Management Services Pty Ltd.

Kase, R. (2023). Polyvagal-informed EMDR: A neuro-informed approach to healing. W. W. Norton & Company.

Knipe, J. (2018). EMDR toolbox: Theory and treatment of complex PTSD and dissociation (2nd ed.). Springer Publishing Company.

Manfield, P., Engel, L., & Greenwald, R. (2017). The flash technique: A rapid method for reducing the emotionality of disturbing memories. Journal of EMDR Practice and Research, 11(4), 195–205. https://doi.org/10.1891/1933-3196.11.4.195

Matthijssen, S. J. M. A., Brouwers, T. C., van den Hout, M. A., & de Jongh, A. (2021). EMDR 2.0: No advantage over standard EMDR in patients with posttraumatic stress disorder and depression. European Journal of Psychotraumatology, 12(1), 1956793.

Shapiro, R. (2005). EMDR solutions: Pathways to healing. W. W. Norton & Company.

Shapiro, R. (Ed.). (2009). EMDR solutions II: For depression, eating disorders, performance, and more. W. W. Norton & Company.

Sheldon, B., & Sheldon, A. (2021). Complex integration of multiple brain systems in therapy. W. W. Norton & Company.

Steele, A. (2020). Developing a secure self: An attachment-based approach to adult psychotherapy. April Steele.

Steele, A. (n.d.). Adventuring spirit. April Steele. https://www.april-steele.ca/product/adventuring-spirit/

Steele, A. (n.d.). Imaginal nurturing. April Steele. https://www.april-steele.ca/product/imaginal-nurturing/

Steele, K., Boon, S., & van der Hart, O. (2016). Treating trauma-related dissociation: A practical, integrative approach. W. W. Norton & Company.

Zimmerman, T. (2024). Four blinks version of flash treatment guide. Four Blinks Version of Flash. https://fourblinks.com/2022/01/20/four-blinks-script/

# Chapter 3

# Attachment-Informed EMDR: Mark Brayne

Mark Brayne, MA, is a psychotherapist, EMDR consultant, and international trainer based in the United Kingdom specializing in attachment-informed EMDR (ai-EMDR). After an early career as a Reuters and BBC foreign correspondent reporting on the Cold War's final years from Moscow, Berlin, Beijing, and London, Mark transitioned to psychotherapy in the 1990s. He first trained in transpersonal psychotherapy before discovering EMDR in 2004.

His journey into trauma work was shaped by both personal and professional experience, and informed by a lifelong interest in language, culture, and human meaning-making. Diagnosed with autism at the age of 70, Mark brings a uniquely structured and nuanced approach to EMDR, integrating attachment theory, developmental neurobiology, and creative imagination into a flexible yet disciplined therapeutic framework.

Mark is also the founder of EMDR Focus in the UK, where he trains clinicians in ai-EMDR, emphasizing intuitive target identification, creative interweaves, and curiosity about how early relational experiences shape nervous system regulation. Drawing on decades of clinical experience, consultation, and supervision, he has developed a distinctive approach grounded in EMDR's standard protocol while expanding its capacity to address complex developmental wounding.

## Which books have influenced your work as a therapist?

***The Road Less Traveled: A New Psychology of Love, Traditional Values, and Spiritual Growth* by M. Scott Peck**

This was the first book to open my eyes to the emotional and spiritual dimensions of healing. In a time of personal crisis, it offered clarity and hope. Peck's description of love as "the will to extend oneself for the purpose of nurturing one's own or another's spiritual growth" resonated deeply. This understanding helped me begin to recognize my attachment patterns and appreciate the central role of relationship, attunement, and repair in emotional well-being. Long before formal training as a therapist, *The Road Less Traveled* planted the seeds that would lead me to EMDR.

***Man and His Symbols* by Carl G. Jung**

This book introduced the significance of the unconscious, archetypes, and the collective symbolic language within us. Jung's focus on dreams, the anima and animus, and the integration of shadow material paralleled my experiences, both personally and professionally. Years later, when I began using EMDR, Jung's concepts helped shape my understanding of the imaginal landscape that is central in attachment-informed processing, where images, symbols, and deep internal narratives transform through reprocessing.

***Goethe's Faust* by Johann Wolfgang von Goethe**

This work has also influenced my understanding of the human experience. Faust's timeless struggle—torn between knowledge and despair on the one hand, and the ache for meaning, love, and integration on the other hand—echoes the internal divisions many clients bring to therapy. The metaphor of "two souls dwelling in one breast" speaks to the divided parts that often emerge during EMDR processing. Faust's redemption through the feminine parallels the essence of attachment repair and emotional healing.

## How do you explain EMDR to your clients?

In my first client conversation, I frame EMDR within an evolutionary and attachment lens. I start, like most therapists, by asking, "How can I help?" As we explore their reasons for seeking therapy, I provide the broader context of how humans are wired to respond to emotional injury.

I explain that, like the body healing physical wounds, our emotional systems are built to process disturbing experiences—though sometimes they get stuck. I describe how unresolved emotional wounds can act like infections: If not addressed, the system struggles to heal. EMDR helps clear these wounds, allowing the natural healing process to resume.

> *Our emotional systems are built to process disturbing experiences—though sometimes they get stuck.*

In practical terms, I introduce clients to the idea that many of today's challenges are rooted in early survival responses that were learned in childhood rarely with conscious awareness. Our nervous system, especially in early development, encodes experiences of connection, safety, and threat long before we have language to describe them. When distressing situations arise later in life, these old survival programs get activated, causing disproportionate emotional reactions in the present.

Often during the first session, to give clients a sense of the process—without actually starting reprocessing—I offer a "psychoeducational bridge." I ask them to recall a recent situation that triggered their distress and then invite them to notice an image, emotion, body sensation, or associated belief that arises. Next, I guide them gently backward. I say, "Connecting with that image, notice what you are feeling and where that's happening in your body. Now, drop back in time, go back as far as you can. Where do you land?" Clients often land in early childhood experiences that can be surprisingly evocative and revealing.

This brief exercise helps clients understand how past experiences shape their present reactions. It reassures them that EMDR addresses the root of their difficulties, not just their symptoms. I explain that while the process can feel intense, we work together at a safe and manageable pace.

Ultimately, I describe EMDR as collaborative, structured, and intuitive—as a way to update the nervous system's old files. This helps clients face challenges with more flexibility, resilience, and peace.

## What advice do you have for new EMDR therapists?

**Stay bold, curious, and true to yourself.** You chose EMDR because you care about healing. You bring clinical experience and your own journey. While EMDR is brilliantly structured, don't let the urge to "get it right" stifle intuition or judgment. The standard protocol works but leaves room for growth and nuance.

Early in my EMDR career, I was anxious about strictly following the standard protocol: identifying the 10 worst memories, rigidly applying NC-PC-VOC-SUD sequences, and staying out of the way in phase 4. Over time, I learned that strict procedural fidelity is not always in the best interest of clients, especially those with complex attachment histories. Our job is not simply to execute a protocol, but to engage with the client's nervous system, their history, and the emotional logic that shaped their survival responses.

**Choose your consultation and supervision carefully.** Work with a consultant who creates space for honest reflection—not someone who leaves you feeling de-skilled or fearful of making mistakes. If you sense that your consultant is more focused on enforcing dogma than helping you build confidence, consider finding someone better suited to your growth. Consultation should feel like a safe space where you can be transparent about what's happening in the room, even when you feel uncertain.

**Record yourself and review your sessions.** You will learn more from watching your own work, including your inevitable missteps, than from many hours of theoretical discussion. Peer review partnerships can be beneficial here: Colleagues willing to offer honest, compassionate feedback will help you refine your attunement, pacing, and presence in the room.

*You will learn more from watching your own work, including your inevitable missteps, than from many hours of theoretical discussion.*

**Remember that perfection is not the goal.** Therapy is a relational, organic, and complex process. Mistakes will happen. What matters most is your capacity to remain present, attuned, and curious—always inviting the client's nervous system to heal in its own time and way.

## What training has had the greatest impact on your practice?

The most transformative shift in my EMDR practice came not through formal training but from a simple handout.

Roughly a decade after completing basic EMDR training, I became an EMDR consultant and integrated much of my earlier background in transpersonal psychotherapy into my work. Like many, I had transitioned from using eye movements to tactile or auditory bilateral stimulation. But I still largely followed the standard protocol, sequencing negative cognitions (NC) and positive cognitions (PC), validity of cognition (VOC) scores, emotions, subjective units of disturbance (SUD), and body as taught.

At the time, many of my clients came through an employee assistance program, which allowed me only five sessions. With such limited time, I couldn't afford to stay out of the way and simply hope for the best. I had to find ways to work efficiently and safely, while still honoring the depth and complexity that clients brought into the room.

The turning point arrived when a consultee returned from a workshop given by Laurel Parnell and showed me a one-page summary of her modified protocol. In place of the more cognitively demanding structure of NC-PC-VOC-emotion-SUD-body, Parnell offered a simplified, attachment-informed alternative: image-emotion-body-belief. Her protocol removed much of the left-brain cognitive load that can destabilize clients early in the process. She also introduced richer resourcing practices, using nurturing, protector, and wise figures alongside the calm place.

By the following week, I was using this approach with every client. The shift was immediate and profound. Clients were more regulated, processing was smoother, and the work often reached developmental roots far more quickly than before. The simplified protocol provided a more intuitive, right brain–friendly approach to activating targets without overwhelming the client's system.

Later, I had the opportunity to train directly with Parnell in group settings and briefly brought her workshops to the UK. While the training itself was valuable, it was really that first exposure—a single piece of paper handed to me by a colleague—that changed my practice overnight.

Since then, I have continued to refine and expand upon these principles, developing the ai-EMDR framework I now teach. It all started with that simple insight: that EMDR can remain firmly grounded in its core principles while allowing for clinical flexibility, attachment focus, and a more intuitive activation of memory networks.

> *EMDR can remain firmly grounded in its core principles while allowing for clinical flexibility, attachment focus, and a more intuitive activation of memory networks.*

## What is one therapeutic approach that integrates really well with EMDR?

While many excellent models integrate well with EMDR, I've found that what matters most is not a specific modality, but the therapist's foundational depth of psychotherapeutic experience, especially when working with complex developmental histories.

In my own work, I draw heavily on my background in transpersonal psychotherapy, which blends psychodynamic, systemic, humanistic, and existential approaches with EMDR's adaptive information processing (AIP) model. This foundation enables me to bring both structure and intuitive flexibility to my work, attuning to the developmental patterns that often underlie adult distress.

Many colleagues highlight Internal Family Systems (IFS) as a complementary approach to EMDR. While IFS offers a helpful language for working with parts, I prefer not to place parts work too rigidly at the center of EMDR sessions. Leading too heavily with parts can bypass the natural unfolding of memory networks that happens when EMDR is grounded in good resourcing and careful target identification. I let parts emerge organically during processing, rather than establishing a fixed map beforehand.

In general, therapists with a strong foundation in psychodynamic, systemic, or transpersonal work are often best equipped to navigate the emotional depth that EMDR can access. Therapists who have undergone their own personal therapy often demonstrate greater attunement, regulation, and capacity for courageous clinical inquiry. By contrast, therapists from strictly cognitive behavioral therapy or medicalized backgrounds may struggle more with the relational and attachment-informed complexities that emerge when processing moves into developmental wounds.

For many clients, dysfunction stems not only from "Big T" trauma, but from the long absence of repair in early attachment relationships. To engage that terrain, EMDR therapists need training that helps them sit in emotional uncertainty, explore relational ruptures, and support the integration of early developmental narratives.

In short, EMDR works best in the hands of therapists with a rich, flexible, and deeply human foundation—and a willingness to keep growing alongside their clients.

> *EMDR works best in the hands of therapists with a rich flexible, and deeply human foundation—and a willingness to keep growing alongside their clients.*

## Which EMDR intervention have you found particularly effective?

Over the past decade, the core ai-EMDR framework I've developed builds on the standard protocol while adapting it to work more directly with developmental and attachment wounds.

At the heart of ai-EMDR is a guiding question: *How did this person come to be the way they are?* Rather than focusing only on specific traumas or events, I work with clients to explore how their nervous system learned to manage life—emotionally, relationally, and behaviorally—through early caregiving experiences, particularly in the relationship with their mother.

The framework retains EMDR's eight-phase structure but includes six attachment-informed modifications, summarized in this mnemonic: Charlie Chaplin Recognizes That Attachments aRe Seriously Salient.

**Charlie Chaplin (Case Conceptualization):** I bring radical curiosity to the client's developmental history, with special attention to survival-driven attachment adaptations rather than only obvious trauma narratives.

**Recognizes (Rich and imaginal resourcing):** In phase 2, I routinely install a full resource team alongside the special/calm place, comprising three nurturing figures, three protector figures, and one wise figure. This strengthens internal self-soothing capacities and activates what Jung called "active imagination," allowing clients to rewire dysfunctional narratives from the past.

**That (Target identification):** I use bridging from present triggers to childhood experiences, often bypassing traditional lists of 10 bad memories and 10 good memories. Instead, we follow present-day activation to its developmental roots.

**Attachments (Appropriate activation):** I simplify phase 3, assessment (which I call "target activation"), to image-emotion- body-belief, without the complete NC-PC-VOC-SUD structure, so the nervous system can engage more intuitively and safely.

**aRe (Reveal, rewire, repair):** In phase 4, while allowing all necessary space for attachment repair to unfold with its own rich imaginal and rewiring arc, I won't hesitate to bring in imaginal interweaves where they're needed to help clients update and repair developmental narratives. This might include curiosity-based inquiry, imaginal rescue, resource figure interventions, and creative narrative rewrites.

> *I won't hesitate to bring in imaginal interweaves where they're needed to help clients update and repair developmental narratives.*

**Seriously Salient (Session Structure):** I structure sessions so that each piece of work feels complete within the time available—returning to present-day relief while tracking how developmental patterns shift as processing unfolds.

Rather than replacing the standard protocol, ai-EMDR works within it, offering a more precise and flexible framework for navigating attachment-informed material. When clients experience these shifts, the results are often striking—not just reduced distress, but greater emotional resilience, intimacy, and self-compassion.

Ultimately, this approach honors EMDR's brilliance while embracing the complexity of human development, helping us move beyond desensitization into the true transformation of the stories our clients carry.

## What role does attachment theory play in your EMDR practice?

In my EMDR practice, attachment theory isn't simply an additional perspective; it's the foundation on which everything else rests. Attachment is not one element among many; it's the organizing principle that shapes how I conceptualize every case, select targets, pace sessions, and navigate the healing process. I would describe my entire approach as attachment-informed EMDR.

Attachment is the lens, and at its core it helps me understand that clients rarely enter therapy solely because of specific "traumas" in the traditional sense. What brings people into therapy are the enduring consequences of how their nervous system learned—always early in life, because that's how it works with mammals—to manage emotional needs, relational ruptures, fear, and unmet longings.

These formative adaptations take place long before cognitive memory develops, rooted in the infant's experience of whether caregivers were available, attuned, responsive, or absent. If they weren't or aren't, or if their presence is emotionally compromised, the infant's nervous system is programmed by evolution to go into survival mode. Without caregiver presence, nurture, and protection, an infant mammal is, after all, lunch to a predator. It's existential.

*Without caregiver presence, nurture, and protection,*
*an infant mammal is, after all, lunch to a predator.*

EMDR's original protocol is brilliantly effective for single-incident traumas. But when we encounter more complex developmental wounding—and we almost always do—the work must adapt to reflect the client's early attachment landscape. It's not simply the bad things that happened, but the absence of repair that matters. The wounds we process are not just about events, but about nervous systems shaped by the root need to self-regulate in the absence of co-regulation.

Attachment informs every stage of my EMDR work. Case conceptualization is a shared journey into how the client's early nervous system learned to survive: flight, fight, freeze, flop, friend, fawn—in that order. Present-day symptoms aren't pathologies, but survival-informed adaptations.

During reprocessing, attachment wounds require active therapeutic presence. While staying out of the way when needed, together with the client, we track the presence of younger ego states—those child parts frozen in time—using creative interweaves, imaginal repair, and relational co-regulation to help them release old survival burdens and integrate into the adult self.

Attachment theory shapes my understanding of healing itself. The goal isn't just desensitization of distress, but the restoration of relational safety—within the client's own system, and often for the first time, with another human being. This is why EMDR, when practiced through an attachment-informed lens, becomes not only technically effective, but also deeply human.

In short, attachment theory is the map, the compass, and the ground beneath my feet in every EMDR session.

## Has a client's cultural background ever influenced your EMDR approach?

One of the privileges of this work is sitting with clients whose personal narratives are profoundly shaped by cultural, historical, and intergenerational layers. A case that stands out involved a client I'll call Amir, a journalist from the Middle East who came to therapy carrying personal trauma and the weight of intergenerational survival.

Amir presented with hyperarousal: insomnia, intrusive images, and a persistent, background sense of dread that no amount of reasoning could resolve. His reporting career exposed him to repeated trauma in conflict zones. But as we explored his history, it became clear that his distress was rooted not just in professional trauma, but in family narratives of displacement, political oppression, and generational loss.

In standard EMDR training, we're taught to focus on discrete events—the 10 worst memories, the "Big T" traumas. With Amir, that approach was far too limited. His anxiety wasn't just a reaction to a few major events; it was an expression of emotional inheritance—unprocessed grief, displacement, and the silent fear passed from parent to child.

> *His anxiety wasn't just a reaction to a few major events;*
> *it was an expression of emotional inheritance.*

Attachment-informed EMDR gave me the flexibility I needed. Rather than start with isolated target memories, I asked Amir to name the felt sense of his distress: chronic vigilance, always watching his back, and the belief that "It's never safe." From there, we used bridging, letting his nervous system take the lead, landing in both childhood and ancestral imagery: stories of exile, forced migration, and oppression that predated his own life.

To stay culturally grounded, I invited Amir to draw on figures from his own tradition for resourcing. His resource team included not just mentors and relatives, but spiritual and historical figures who embodied strength, wisdom, and protection—in ways that felt deeply meaningful to him. These imaginal supports became powerful anchors during processing.

In phase 4, when early memories of helplessness surfaced, I used interweaves that honored both the personal and the collective. I said, "Let your ancestors witness how far you've come," or "Let those who came before you stand behind you now." These interventions helped his system process both personal fear and inherited narratives.

This case deepened my understanding of how trauma rarely exists in isolation. Cultural and intergenerational forces are often woven into symptoms in ways that can't be separated from the individual's story. EMDR—especially when practiced with flexibility and cultural humility—enables us to work at multiple levels, acknowledging the full complexity of the human experience.

Since Amir, I approach each client with a deeper awareness of what lives not just in their personal biography, but in their cultural bloodstream—and of how EMDR can update not only their nervous system, but the echoes of generations past.

> *I approach each client with a deeper awareness of what lives not just in their personal biography, but in their cultural bloodstream.*

## What EMDR success story caught you by surprise?

One client story that stays with me involved a woman I'll call Joan, a highly capable professional in her early 50s who had long struggled with anxiety, intrusive nightmares, and a pervasive fear of emotional messiness, both in herself and in others.

The breakthrough began not with a traumatic memory, but with a dream. She described waking in terror from an image of wiping red pepper seeds from her burned wrists—vivid, disturbing, and powerfully symbolic. A few days earlier, she had indeed burned her hands while cooking. The dream's intensity, however, pointed to something more profound.

Rather than analyzing the dream cognitively, we used it as a spontaneous entry point for EMDR processing. As Joan focused on the image, I invited her to drop back in time using a bridge. I said, "Staying with that image, that emotion, that body sensation, and the belief about yourself [which was, 'I can't bear mess'], drop back in time. Go back as far as you can. First place you land." What surfaced was a deeply embedded childhood pattern: her mother's obsessive and ongoing intolerance for anything messy—emotional, relational, or physical.

In Joan's early years, any expression of distress or untidiness was met with maternal disapproval, withdrawal, or subtle shaming. Over time, she internalized a fierce pressure to contain and sanitize all emotional experiences, which later manifested as hypervigilance, self-criticism, and difficulty tolerating vulnerability, especially in relationships.

We processed these early attachment wounds scene by scene, as if for real, and used imaginary interweaves, resource figures, and eventually her own adult self to offer the comfort and acceptance she never received. Joan's nervous system began to soften. The nightmares stopped. Her anxiety diminished. Most strikingly, she began to tolerate—and even welcome—emotional vulnerability in herself and in close relationships.

What surprised me most was how profoundly her system responded—not to revisiting specific traumas, but to giving the exiled child part of herself the experience of being welcomed, messy and all. The dream had distilled her survival strategy into a single haunting image. EMDR, used intuitively and with creative imagination, allowed her nervous system to rewrite that early story in ways years of insight-oriented therapy never had.

Joan's story illustrates the power of attachment-informed EMDR. Often what drives dysfunction isn't what happened, but what should have happened and didn't—the absence of repair, attunement, and emotional permission in early life. When we access those deeper developmental layers, the results can be quietly, sometimes dramatically, transformative.

> *Often what drives dysfunction isn't what happened,*
> *but what should have happened but didn't.*

## How has your approach to EMDR evolved since you first completed your training?

When I first trained in EMDR, I followed the standard protocol almost religiously. Like most of us, I was taught to identify 10 worst memories, select the target, run through the NC-PC-VOC-SUDs-body sequence, and stay out of the way during processing. The training provided a brilliant structure, and I remain deeply grateful to Francine Shapiro for creating that framework. Still, even in those early days, something about the rigid application of the protocol didn't always sit comfortably, especially when I was face-to-face with real clients.

The turning point came as I began working with more complex clients whose struggles were rooted not in isolated traumas, but in early attachment disruptions and developmental wounds. Many couldn't identify their worst memories. Their trauma lived not in events, but in years of emotional absence, misattunement, and unmet needs. Staying strictly within the standard protocol often left them dysregulated, looping, or unable to engage.

Over time, my approach evolved into what I now describe as attachment-informed EMDR. I still honor the eight phases and three-pronged structure of EMDR, but I've adapted how I work with target identification, resourcing, activation, and structure.

Where I once sought isolated traumatic events, I now focus on patterns of survival learning—how the client's nervous system learned to manage life from its earliest experiences. I use bridging to track present-day triggers back to their developmental origins, uncovering memories the client had often not consciously recalled before.

As I've outlined elsewhere, and with thanks to Laurel Parnell for mainstreaming it, I've also expanded resourcing beyond the basic calm place. I now always, and with every client, tap in (a better term than "install") a whole resource team—nurturers, protectors, and wise figures—to prepare for deeper, safer work with attachment wounds.

In processing, interweaves and creative imagination are my essential tools for working with root experiences. I've never resonated with the generic term "cognitive interweaves." Anything the therapist does, or indeed *is*, is an interweave. Cognitive interweaves are just one kind of intervention. So I tend to be more active and structured than many EMDR trainers—staying out of the way when needed, but always working explicitly with the adult client to engage with and proactively revise their early stories.

My favorite metaphor is the time-traveling DeLorean from *Back to the Future*. I'm the driver, and the client's adult self is the navigator. Clients from the broadest range of cultures recognize the film, and it offers a playful, poignant frame for revisiting childhood and changing the outcome. I even show them my 2,000-piece LEGO DeLorean—a gift from my family, painstakingly assembled in the post-Christmas quiet. The metaphor often sets the tone for surprisingly powerful work.

So, what's changed? My trust in EMDR's flexibility—and my confidence that courage, structure, focus, and attunement matter more than rigid fidelity. What hasn't changed is my awe at the core of this work: bilateral stimulation unlocking the nervous system's deep, evolutionary drive to heal.

> *Courage, structure, focus, and attunement matter more than rigid fidelity.*

## What self-care practices do you engage in regularly?

Long-distance cycling is my anchor. Each year, I carve out time to ride—often for weeks at a stretch—usually with my partner on our sturdy tandem bike. These breaks help both me and my clients pause, reflect, and integrate. My partner and I have ridden 2,000 miles the length of New Zealand, 3,500 miles around Germany, and 2,500 miles through France. We've even pedaled through the Russian enclave of Kaliningrad on our way from Warsaw, Poland, to Tallinn, Estonia.

Cycling functions for me like an EMDR-informed retreat: a steady rhythm, bilateral stimulation, and long stretches of silence. On a tandem bike, there's also the added rhythm of conversation—front captain and rear stoker—which seems to mirror the bilateral back-and-forth of therapy itself.

> *Cycling functions for me like an EMDR-informed retreat: a steady rhythm, bilateral stimulation, and long stretches of silence.*

While I also enjoy walks in the woods and quiet moments, I recharge through learning. I find comfort in studying languages, Russian and Hungarian, most recently, and even in following international news, perhaps a vestige of my journalism days. It might not be traditional self-care, but staying informed grounds me in the world.

Finally, I make space for peer consultation, personal therapy when needed, and time with two small grandchildren—we're fortunate to have them—as well as blocks of time away from screens and professional demands. The work we do invites us deeply into other people's nervous systems. Self-care is what allows me to stay grounded enough to meet them there.

## References

Goethe, J. W. von. (2008). Faust: Part one (D. Luke, Trans.). Oxford University Press.

Jung, C. G., von Franz, M.-L., Henderson, J. L., Jacobi, J., & Jaffé, A. (1964). Man and his symbols. Doubleday.

Peck, M. S. (2003). The road less traveled, timeless edition: A new psychology of love, traditional values and spiritual growth. Touchstone. (Original work published 1978)

Shapiro, F. (2017). Eye movement desensitization and reprocessing (EMDR) therapy: Basic principles, protocols, and procedures (3rd ed.). Guilford Press.

# Chapter 4

# Nature-Based Diversity: Jennifer Marchand

Rooted in Canada's vibrant Acadian community, Jennifer Marchand, MA, CCC, RCAT, CCTP-II, grew up seeing the impacts of rural poverty. Also witness to her grandmother's years of institutionalization—due to misdiagnosis and severe mistreatment of trauma—Jennifer felt impelled to support those affected by adversity, especially in low-resource settings and within marginalized communities.

As a Canadian Certified Counsellor, a certified trauma specialist, and an EMDRIA-approved consultant, Jennifer carries a deep commitment to nature-based practices. She has worked for more than a decade in non-Western contexts and Indigenous communities, and has training in Indigenous Focusing-Oriented Therapy (IFOT). Jennifer blends EMDR with ecotherapy and the creative arts. Her career has taken her to Vietnam, Kurdistan, Afghanistan, and now Ethiopia, where she lives with her husband and two children. Across all these settings, her approach to trauma therapy remains shaped by cross-cultural exchange, community, and the healing power of the natural world.

## Which books have influenced your work as a therapist?

### *Anti-Racist Psychotherapy: Confronting Systemic Racism and Healing Racial Trauma* by David Archer

This book offers a framework for acknowledging and addressing racial trauma. Archer argues that, for too long, Eurocentric models of mental health have overlooked or minimized the impacts of systemic racism. As EMDR therapists, many of us haven't been given the tools to meaningfully integrate racial, historical, and generational trauma into our formulations or treatment plans. Archer fills that gap beautifully.

His book centers the voices and lived experiences of Black, Indigenous, and other racialized clients, which helps therapists—especially those without this lived experience, such as myself—broaden our understanding of racism as a form of psychological violence and trauma. He blends anti-oppressive theory, neuroscience, and trauma-informed practice in a way that supports clients in healing from racial trauma and reclaiming identity, dignity, and agency.

Many therapists are familiar with trauma-informed care, which helped us move past the question "What's wrong with you?" and toward asking, "What happened to you?" Building on this, Archer invites us to go further by asking, "What systems and societal forces have shaped and impacted you?" This deepens our understanding of how societal forces shape suffering and why they must be named.

As a consultant, I know many EMDR therapists are hesitant to address social and cultural identities in the therapy space. But to do so—with humility and curiosity—is to create space for racial trauma, oppression, and discrimination to be named and brought into the healing process. It also requires ongoing work around anti-oppression and privilege—and a willingness to challenge, rather than reenact, the ways racism is embedded in the mental health field.

> *Create space for racial trauma, oppression, and discrimination to be named and brought into the healing process.*

***Cultural Humility in Art Therapy* by Louvenia C. Jackson**

Building on these ideas, and as an art therapist, I highly recommend this book to EMDR therapists. Cultural humility is not just a concept; it's a living, embodied practice. Jackson offers creative, practical tools to help therapists reflect on their own identities, biases, and power dynamics. Through art directives and case examples, she shows how creativity can open space for difficult conversations around race and identity in clinical work.

***What My Bones Know: A Memoir of Healing from Complex Trauma* by Stephanie Foo**

Foo's account of living with complex and attachment trauma is personal, raw, and beautifully told. It carries a clear message: Healing is possible. As trauma therapists, we sometimes need that reminder so we can hold hope for our clients too.

Foo's lived experience of generational and immigrant trauma also sheds light on the invisible pressures many clients face—and the importance of helping them name and explore those experiences. I've recommended this book to many clients—especially complex trauma survivors—as a way to cultivate self-compassion and recognize how life experiences beyond their control shape functioning and well-being. Foo's voice offers a powerful psychoeducational tool, helping clients understand the lasting psychological wounds of chronic "little t" trauma.

These books can support EMDR therapists in cultivating curiosity, humility, and openness—while honoring the full complexity of each client's healing journey.

## How do you explain EMDR to your clients?

Explaining EMDR and its treatment steps to clients in a way that makes sense to them is not an easy task, especially when we ourselves do not fully understand why it is so effective. Therapists often struggle to apply the concepts and language they learned in basic training to their work with clients. I think the "weird factor" of EMDR leads many new practitioners to overexplain the process using neuroscientific terms and concepts as a way to legitimize the use of eye movements, which can both overwhelm or disinterest the client.

Also, EMDR is not a self-explanatory acronym. If someone were to ask me what EMDR is, and I responded with, "eye movement desensitization and reprocessing," I wouldn't blame them for looking at me sideways. I have found it helpful to keep things simple, especially during the preparation phase. It can sound overly clinical or abstract at first, so I like to use a mix of metaphors and visual resources to break it down in a way that makes sense to clients, resonates with them, and helps them feel like an active and equal part of the process.

Here's a helpful alliteration I use to explain the acronym and orient clients to how EMDR works:

- ***E** is for an eight-phase, evidence-based, and experiential approach to trauma* *recovery. It's based on years of research and broken down into steps that I'll guide you through. It's something we do together, not just talk therapy.*

- ***M** is for metabolizing unprocessed memories through mindful noticing and movement, such as tapping or eye movements. This helps the brain make new meaning of the past.*
- ***D** is for distracting the mind while thinking about something upsetting, a phenomenon known as "dual attention." One part of your brain focuses on the memory while another stays anchored in the present.*
- ***R** is for reprocessing. We can't change the past, but we can change our relationship to it. This process helps let go of beliefs that were left behind, strengthens your sense of worth, and clears the blocks that keep you stuck.*

## What advice do you have for new EMDR therapists?

**Don't underestimate the importance of phase 2.** I encourage my consultees to spend time building up adaptive information so the client's brain has something helpful to connect with during reprocessing. Without enough adaptive memory, the stuck material has nowhere to go. For example, if a client has no lived experience of safety, how can they resolve memories rooted in fear or violation? We are looking for what heals as much as we are looking for what hurts.

> *We are looking for what heals as much as we are looking for what hurts.*

Preparation means helping clients access internal and external resources: strengths, skills, qualities, support systems, updated perspectives, self-worth, and compassion. These can be installed and strengthened using present-moment awareness, somatic cues, and bilateral stimulation. If a client can't access a calm memory, we create calm together in the session using music, drawing, movement, or YouTube videos, then install those experiences using bilateral stimulation (BLS).

If a client has never felt validated, offer that in the therapeutic relationship. Many people don't know what it feels like to be respected. When your client sets a boundary, communicates a need, says no without consequences, or shares something shameful and isn't met with judgment, those are all new experiences.

Slow down and highlight how these moments are different. Invite your client to notice the change and feel it in their body. Then use BLS to install it—perhaps using words like, "I can learn to express my needs." These micromoments lay the groundwork for healing interpersonal trauma. They become adaptive information—new, corrective experiences the brain can draw on to resolve older wounds.

Look for "glimmers," not just triggers. A term coined by Deb Dana, glimmers refer to small moments of safety, connection, or joy that help clients return to a state of regulation. They might be a scent, a hobby, a tree, a pet, or a memory of feeling capable or connected. These can be installed as resources to support both stabilization and reprocessing.

**Find positive goals that move the work forward.** Clients often express goals in negative terms: "I want to stop yelling" or "I don't want to feel anxious." Our role is to help them turn those into positive, forward-moving goals. I often ask, "If you weren't doing that, what would you be doing instead?" This reveals something more meaningful to work toward—a reason to keep going when the work gets hard.

Without a clear goal, trauma work can feel like suffering without purpose. When consultees feel stuck or as if they're working harder than the client, I ask, "What makes this work worth it for them?" Often, we realize this step was skipped. Clients need to see EMDR as part of a larger plan for change.

*Without a clear goal, trauma work*
*can feel like suffering without purpose.*

**Cluster memories to make the work manageable.** Memories don't always present themselves as a single event. With complex trauma, memories often form clusters—ongoing experiences like neglect, bullying, discrimination, repeated surgeries, or abuse. When a client says something happened "a lot" or "over time," help them map the start and end. Sometimes it's still ongoing, so the "end" may be in the future.

Other clusters involve separate but similar events, such as different car accidents or assaults. Mapping them helps clarify how many times something occurred and when.

You can then target the first, worst, and most recent events to get the full arc. This makes reprocessing more efficient and often leads to generalization across the network.

Grouping memories into clusters helps clients work through their past in a manageable way. It gives structure to the work and allows them to experience progress without getting overwhelmed.

## What is one therapeutic approach that integrates really well with EMDR?

I am passionate about using nature-based metaphors to offer an organic, supportive, and nonpathologizing way to engage clients in therapy. One example is introducing clients to a nature-based understanding of parts from the Internal Family Systems (IFS) model. I am level 2–trained in IFS and find that it integrates smoothly with the EMDR protocol. Integrating IFS into the preparation phase enables clients to notice and relate to their internal experiences with curiosity and compassion—skills essential for EMDR success.

I introduce clients to IFS by describing the internal world as an ecosystem that requires various elements to function and remain balanced. These elements are like "parts," each with its own roles, beliefs, feelings, memories, and origins. In IFS, some parts are "protectors" that shield us from pain and vulnerability. Others, called "exiles," hold emotional wounds pushed out of awareness. At the core is "Self-energy," a calm, wise, and compassionate inner force that helps all parts feel seen, safe, and supported.

Instead of using IFS terms like "firefighters" and "managers," I describe protector parts as clouds and wind, exiles as seedlings, and Self-energy as the sun. This framework is often more accessible and culturally adaptable. Manager parts are like clouds that keep the exile from surfacing by covering the sky and blocking emotions and sensations, instead focusing on perfectionism, overworking, or people-pleasing. This dampens joy and vitality, creating a dull, overcast quality in daily life, in exchange for a sense of safety.

> *I describe protector parts as clouds and wind,*
> *exiles as seedlings, and Self-energy as the sun.*

Firefighter parts are like winds that blow in when the exile, or emerging seedling, begins to surface. These winds create chaos or distraction to quickly bury the exile, such as through substance use, risk-taking, self-harm, or outbursts. The winds and clouds develop their own push-and-pull dynamic within the ecosystem. Winds can blow clouds away, leaving them fearful of losing control and more critical of impulsive, chaotic behaviors.

Exiles are like seedlings buried under the soil. These vulnerable parts long for healing and connection but are blocked from the sun's warmth and nutrients. Often young, they can bring joy and vitality if they release their burdens, like a seedling shedding its seed coat, and receive the healing rays of Self-energy. Like the sun, Self-energy offers warmth, nurturance, and healing to all parts. Clearing the clouds and calming the wind allows the seedling to emerge and thrive.

During EMDR preparation, I guide clients through this metaphor to help them recognize internal patterns as protective strategies that conceal pain and vulnerability. I might ask, "What behaviors help you cloud over so you don't have to feel emotions, stay in control, numb out, or stay focused on tasks?" Or "Can you recall reactions that blow in suddenly like gusts of wind—fast, impulsive behaviors that feel chaotic or out of control, often in response to something upsetting? These can quickly push the pain back under the surface so you regain control."

As clients see that their system is reenacting survival patterns, they develop self-compassion and ways to soothe and update their protectors. When these parts feel seen and reassured that the trauma is past, they often soften. This creates space for reprocessing the wounds exiles carry. Integrating this nature-based IFS approach into EMDR preparation helps clients stabilize, observe patterns with less shame, reassure their inner parts, and access their Self-energy, allowing their inner sun to offer compassion, nurturance, and protection throughout the ecosystem.

*As clients see that their system is reenacting survival patterns, they develop self-compassion and ways to soothe and update their protectors.*

## What role does attachment theory play in your EMDR practice?

When working with clients who have attachment trauma, effective attachment resourcing must come first. Without it, there is no available adaptive information to support healing.

At the same time, this resourcing can be challenging because it often stirs memories of missing experiences or abuse and neglect. To address both needs, I developed a protocol that combines resourcing and reprocessing simultaneously, using nature-based materials in a safe, grounded, and contained way.

The Resource Place protocol invites clients to use a small seed, bean, or grain of rice to represent the beginning of their life. This object is sensory, tangible, and symbolic, helping clients connect with nonverbal parts of their story in a grounded and contained way.

Clients first create a nurturing "resource place" for their seed using art and natural materials. This becomes a visual representation of safety, nurturance, and potential for growth, similar to a womb.

From there, we move through developmental periods, starting with conception, and scan each stage. Any discomfort or distress that arises is reprocessed as a target memory. Clients do not need to recall specific events from early years. Instead, they notice images, sensations, or emotions that arise. This work is about tuning into what is held in the body and imagination, then engaging gently with what emerges.

We then bring the positive cognition, installed in phase 5, back to the "resource place" to reinforce new adaptive beliefs. Clients may write them down or represent them symbolically. This process is repeated until the distressing implicit information from the preverbal years has been combed through and cleared.

Over time, this process lays a stronger foundation for later reprocessing. The Resource Place protocol, strengthened with positive cognitions, becomes a grounding and nurturing internal space clients can return to repeatedly. This protocol is described in detail in *Ecotherapy-Informed EMDR*, which includes a step-by-step script and a case example featuring Noriko Baba, a skilled therapist and friend.

## Has a client's cultural background ever influenced your EMDR approach?

Many traditions around the world view wellness as a state of harmony and balance in our relationships with community, nature, and the spiritual world. In contrast, Eurocentric and Western approaches often frame psychological distress through a narrow, biomedical lens, using reductionist cognitive models that focus on individual symptoms. They often overlook the body, as well as interconnectedness with relationships and surrounding systems.

I am passionate about making EMDR more culturally responsive by integrating an ecocentric lens that honors our place in the natural world. This brings us back to our bodies, to each other, and to the healing power of deep connection with nature. For example, Africentric healing frameworks, as described by David Archer in *Racial Trauma Recovery*, emphasize that imbalance in our relationship with nature and spirit contributes to emotional and psychological distress. In many Indigenous communities, healing is about restoring harmony with oneself, others, the land, ancestors, and the cosmos. Drawing on Judith L. Herman's seminal *Trauma and Recovery: The Aftermath of Violence*, we must also view healing as a relational process.

> *In many Indigenous communities, healing is about restoring harmony with oneself, others, the land, ancestors, and the cosmos.*

Integrating nature-based metaphors and materials into EMDR has been one of the primary ways I make it more culturally responsive for the individuals and communities I serve. Ecocentric, embodied, and relational practices are often experienced by clients as deeply human and culturally respectful.

The three-pronged protocol—which targets the past, present, and future—is essential to effective trauma treatment. However, the word "pronged" can sound rigid, like the tines of a fork. In contrast, many cultures view time as fluid and interconnected rather than linear or fixed. To reflect this, I use nature-based and culturally relevant metaphors to explain the flow of EMDR. They also explain how working with all strands of past, present, and future experiences can help resolve and integrate memories while also weaving in and strengthening resources.

These micromoments lay the groundwork for healing interpersonal trauma by providing adaptive information—new, corrective experiences that the nervous system can store alongside the original memory, transforming its emotional impact.

Here are a few metaphors I use that make the three-pronged protocol and the rationale behind treatment plans more accessible and meaningful for clients.

- **The river:** A river represents how we can access different points in time: past (upstream), present (the current), and future (downstream). This metaphor supports a fluid, nonlinear understanding of healing, where we can revisit what needs attention and move with the current of the process. All branches of a river are interconnected and affect each other, flowing together and intersecting at different points. Past work affects the present and the future.

- **The *sankofa*:** The West African Akan symbol *sankofa* depicts a bird turning back to retrieve an egg from its back. The word means "go back and get it" in Twi. I first encountered the symbol while studying sub-Saharan African art history in Ghana during an undergraduate exchange. Later, in Ethiopia, I began using it to explain the three-pronged protocol. It reflects the EMDR stance of standing in the present while reaching back to heal the past and bringing forward the resources and wisdom from that time, represented by the egg. This honors a client's culture, traditions, and ancestral knowledge, using the past as a resource for the healing journey ahead.

- **The braid:** A braid weaves together three strands, just as EMDR weaves together past, present, and future. Braids appear in many cultures: in hair, textiles, and natural materials such as sweetgrass. In many Indigenous communities in North America, braiding sweetgrass is a sacred and ceremonial process. Like a braid, EMDR weaves time strands together to create new meaning, resilience, and integration.

- **The triquetra knot:** The ancient Celtic triquetra symbolizes the interconnection of time, as well as the connection between earth, sea, and sky, and body, mind, and spirit. The knot is seamless and unbroken. In EMDR, we move between the loops of past, present, and future to help restore harmony and balance.

## How has your approach to EMDR evolved since you first completed your training?

Over the years, my EMDR work has evolved by weaving core concepts with nature-based metaphors. These images help EMDR feel more organic, intuitive, and familiar, especially in diverse cultural contexts.

Ecotherapy-informed EMDR reframes the standard eight phases and key components, including the adaptive information processing (AIP) model, through a nature-based lens, offering a grounded and intuitive way for therapists and clients to understand EMDR.

## The Internal River Metaphor

At the heart of EMDR is the AIP model. Francine Shapiro described a natural brain-body system that processes life experiences. When something overwhelming happens, this system can get blocked, leaving the memory stuck in its original state—images, emotions, sensations, and beliefs intact.

I describe the AIP system as an internal river—a current carrying experiences toward integration and resolution. When it flows freely, we take in the good, release what no longer serves us, and move forward. But when something heavy drops in, like trauma, it blocks the flow. Pileups form, leading to "flooding" or "drought" (anxiety, overwhelm, dysregulation).

EMDR helps us "travel upstream" to identify and dislodge blockages, allowing them to be carried forward. With bilateral stimulation—such as eye movements or tapping—the stuck material shifts. Emotional charge fades, and sharp edges smooth, like rocks tumbling, until the memory is integrated and no longer raw.

The internal river metaphor reinforces that healing is already within the client—waiting to be unblocked.

> *The internal river metaphor reinforces that healing is already within the client—waiting to be unblocked.*

## The Mountain Metaphor

The river metaphor helps clients and consultees understand integration, while the mountain illustrates the reprocessing journey. Like mountains, trauma memories can feel intimidating, but healing happens when we return to the place where the mountain was formed. I explain reprocessing as a journey through the mountain, starting at the peak—the worst part. From there, clients gain perspective, identifying beliefs, emotions, and body sensations—in the assessment phase. At the peak, they describe what they see, feel, and believe.

Then we journey up and down. The client is the "pathfinder." They choose the route, and we follow. I trust that the path holds information, and I guide only if they get stuck or overwhelmed.

My role is to facilitate movement with dual-attention stimulus, helping the client process what emerges. We pause between sets, notice what arises, and follow their next steps. As they descend, they revisit aspects of memory with present awareness, gather resources, and shift perspectives—what Shapiro calls the "progressive stages of self-healing." We follow until the memory feels complete at the mountain's base.

We repeat the climb as needed for peace and resolution, checking the peak for any new material before ending the journey.

This process changes the client's relationship to the memory. The mountain remains but loses its charge. New paths are cleared, unneeded elements eroded. Once traversed, the memory no longer holds power—it rests in the past.

*The mountain remains but loses its charge. New paths are cleared, unneeded elements eroded.*

I explore this framework further in my book, *Ecotherapy-Informed EMDR: A Holistic and Creative Approach to Providing Culturally Responsive Trauma Treatment*, wherein I embed the eight phases of the standard protocol. It helps me explain EMDR more intuitively to clients and guide consultees in navigating the protocol.

I might ask, "Where are you with your client—on or off the mountain?" or "What will help them feel ready to journey through that memory?" The metaphor reinforces that reprocessing happens on the mountain, and we must come fully off—out of the memory—to contain, stabilize, and ground.

## References

Archer, D. (2022). Racial trauma recovery: A practical guide to addressing racial trauma in psychotherapy. PESI Publishing.

Archer, D. (2021). Anti-racist psychotherapy: Confronting systemic racism and healing racial trauma. Each One Teach One Publications.

Dana, D. (2023). Anchored: How to befriend your nervous system using polyvagal theory. Sounds True.

Foo, S. (2022). What my bones know: A memoir of healing from complex trauma. Ballantine Books.

Herman, J. L. (1992). Trauma and recovery: The aftermath of violence—from domestic abuse to political terror. Basic Books.

Jackson, L. C. (2020). Cultural humility in art therapy: Applications for practice, research, social justice, self-care, and pedagogy. Jessica Kingsley Publishers.

Marchand, J. (2025). Ecotherapy-informed EMDR: A holistic and creative approach to providing culturally responsive trauma treatment. PESI Publishing.

Schwartz, R. C. (1995). Internal family systems therapy. Guilford Press.

Shapiro, F. (2018). Eye movement desensitization and reprocessing (EMDR) therapy: Basic principles, protocols, and procedures (3rd ed.). Guilford Press.

Turcotte, S., & Schiffer, J. J. (2014). Aboriginal/Indigenous focusing-oriented therapy. In G. Madison (Ed.), Emerging practice in focusing-oriented psychotherapies: Innovative theory and application (pp. 55–74). Jessica Kingsley Publishers.

# Chapter 5

# The Slow, Nonlinear Path: Thomas Zimmerman

Thomas Zimmerman, MSEd, LPCC, is an EMDRIA-approved consultant and trainer. He lives and practices in the Cleveland, Ohio, area and is the author of *EMDR with Complex Trauma*. Thomas developed the Four Blinks Version of Flash, a variation of the Flash technique tailored specifically for individuals with complex trauma. He has trained tens of thousands of therapists worldwide in trauma-focused care.

## Which books have influenced your work as a therapist?

***A Therapist's Guide to EMDR* by Laurel Parnell**

I encountered this book between part I and part II trainings, and it was exactly the refresher I needed to deepen my understanding of EMDR therapy and grasp the purpose of each phase more clearly. While I have since come to appreciate the main Shapiro text, I remember thinking at the time, *This is the book I wish Francine Shapiro had written about EMDR therapy.... It's clear, practical, and written from a place of passion for this work.*

This is also the book I've had the hardest time keeping in my library, as I loan out copies to newly trained friends and coworkers, and they are rarely returned. I get it—it's hard to return a book that you might need later that day.

***Attachment-Focused EMDR* by Laurel Parnell**

My first encounter with this book came at a time of urgent clinical need, several months after completing part II training. I had clients who were consistently getting stuck in attachment-wound memories, and every attempt to help unstick them using standard cognitive interweaves was ineffective.

Worse still, standard closure strategies failed to release the tension in the parts of them that were most activated. Some of these clients reported significant decompensation between sessions, as though they had hooked onto a whale during the session and were still being dragged along for days afterward.

Helping these clients develop and practice attachment-figure resources allowed them to conclude these difficult, attachment-focused sessions with greater safety and grounding. The attachment resources also helped them develop some of the adaptive information they were missing.

## What is your approach to addressing ambivalence or hesitation when introducing EMDR to clients?

The more I work with clients who have complex trauma, the less useful I find the word "resistance." Many clients have long-standing survival strategies that pull them in the opposite direction of where I'm trying to guide them. They've survived by avoiding their trauma because very little of their trauma-related activation has ever led to something productive.

> *The more I work with clients who have complex trauma, the less useful I find the word "resistance."*

EMDR therapy asks clients to slow down, be present, and notice. Many have survived by doing the opposite—not slowing down, not being present, and staying ahead of it.

It's often helpful to remind clients that EMDR therapy is different from other therapies. It works precisely because it's different. I may ask clients to do things that feel nonintuitive or even weird. If it feels like too much, we can dip our toes in—we don't have to jump into the deep end.

Many traditional mindfulness approaches are designed for relatively healthy clients. When working with the nervous systems of clients with complex trauma, we should expect resourcing to be slow, require significant modifications, and be tailored to the unique system in front of us.

## What advice do you have for new EMDR therapists?

**Learn by doing.** Learning EMDR therapy isn't all that different from learning anything else as a therapist. You'll get better by doing a lot of it—from a place of curiosity and compassion. Few practitioners continue to use EMDR regularly a year after training. My hope is that, with ongoing support, you will remain committed to the therapy in the long term—for the benefit of both you and your clients.

**Apply insights thoughtfully and adapt to each case.** It's essential to learn from the lessons EMDR therapy offers with complex clients, but avoid overgeneralizing.

**Understand that EMDR therapy with complex clients is especially challenging.** Almost all work with these clients is hard. This difficulty is not a reflection of your ability. Success requires learning strategies that go beyond basic training, as foundational skills are often designed for healthier populations, whom you'll encounter less often.

**Be ready to work with clients who cannot tolerate activation.** EMDR therapy requires clients to have the capacity to activate in moderation, slow down, stay present, and notice sensations they've likely spent much of their lives avoiding. You'll work with clients who are phobic of slowing down, being present, and noticing. EMDR therapy is a difficult clinical task—even for those of us who've done this work across thousands of sessions—especially with clients who most need to heal. With complex clients, EMDR therapy is not a magic wand. Without enough adaptive information, there may not be any magic in it at all.

*With complex clients, EMDR therapy is not a magic wand. Without enough adaptive information, there may not be any magic in it at all.*

## What is one therapeutic approach that integrates really well with EMDR?

Parts work, in all its varieties, integrates well with EMDR therapy. I often incorporate parts work in phase 2 to help clients develop and strengthen essential adaptive information they may have missed during childhood. Many clients with complex trauma have highly conflicted internal parts systems. The more adult parts may shame, blame, judge, and humiliate the younger parts for not making "good" decisions.

A lot of healing happens through a bridge of empathy between parts. All healing in EMDR therapy occurs across a discrepancy of information; distressing learning must connect with sufficient adaptive learning to be metabolized. You cannot connect a lie to a lie in EMDR therapy, nor can you connect a lie to nothing.

*You cannot connect a lie to a lie in EMDR therapy, nor can you connect a lie to nothing.*

We develop adaptive information experientially. We are wounded experientially, we resource experientially, and we heal experientially. Parts work allows aspects of ourselves to have relational experiences with one another that differ from those learned in traumatic situations. For many of my clients, parts work marks the beginning of self-listening, self-understanding, and self-compassion. It is also the beginning of more effective self-management. Parts work helps clients develop and experience the very adaptive information they most lacked in childhood.

Parts work alone can be healing. It's one of the few approaches that helps clients develop the core adaptive information needed to resolve their deepest wounds.

## Have you experienced imposter syndrome?

It's not unusual for me to feel confused during a client's reprocessing session—even after conducting roughly 10,000 of them. As a guide, I sometimes give incorrect guidance. And yes, sometimes I make the same mistake more than once. I can promise you that no one is doing perfect EMDR with clients who have complex trauma.

This work is always slow. It is rarely linear. Case conceptualization unfolds gradually, and when healing comes, it often comes slowly. Blind curves are normal. As trauma therapists, we walk mostly blind through the nervous systems of others. We will misstep. If something is inevitable, it must also, somehow, be okay. When clients struggle, that is not failure; it's information. Often, it's vital guidance for the work ahead.

*When clients struggle, that is not failure; it's information.*

You probably worked for months or years with clients with complex trauma before you were trained in EMDR therapy. Of all the professionals in the world, you know what complex trauma looks like. You know what a bad idea looks like. You've likely spent more face-to-face time with clients with complex trauma than with your own partners, friends, or family. Let everything you know about complex trauma shape how you conduct EMDR therapy—not the other way around.

It's important to dig deep and find ways to do this work, despite its difficulties. It's the heart of your job. You are a trauma therapist, and your clients urgently need to heal. Throughout much of human history, most people died with their nervous systems still carrying their traumatic load. Through all the wars, toxic dynamics, and epidemics, humans have had the capacity to heal themselves. We now know multiple ways humans can heal. EMDR therapy is one of them. And you are trained in it. If you need help, there are many people available to assist you.

## What self-care practices do you engage in regularly?

Many EMDR therapists are trained in versions of the Flash technique. Unlike EMDR therapy, most people can easily use Flash in a self-administered way and resolve issues safely, predictably, and pleasantly. It has become my go-to mindfulness strategy. You can do Flash while walking, petting a dog, bathing, watching television, or even eating pizza. Flash can potentially turn any pleasant activity into a transformational trauma therapy.

Flash is an excellent self-care strategy for those working with particularly challenging clients. Clients who activate our own issues bring valuable information about our nervous systems—assuming we're actively engaging in our own healing and development. Flash is also an excellent self-care tool for relational triggers, whether you're living with teenagers or a partner who occasionally tests your patience.

Flash can be especially helpful if you work in an agency where organizational goals don't always align with what you and your clients need to survive and thrive.

## References

Manfield, P., Lovett, J., Engel, L., & Manfield, D. (2017). Use of the flash technique in EMDR therapy: Four case examples. Journal of EMDR Practice and Research, 11(4), 195–205. https://doi.org/10.1891/1933-3196.11.4.195

Parnell, L. (2007). A therapist's guide to EMDR: Tools and techniques for successful treatment. W. W. Norton & Company.

Parnell, L. (2013). Attachment-focused EMDR: Healing relational trauma. W. W. Norton & Company.

Shapiro, F. (2018). Eye movement desensitization and reprocessing (EMDR) therapy: Basic principles, protocols, and procedures (3rd ed.). Guilford Press.

Zimmerman, T. (2024a). EMDR with complex trauma. EMDR Training Collaborative.

Zimmerman, T. (2024b). Four blinks version of flash treatment guide. Four Blinks Version of Flash. https://fourblinks.com/2022/01/20/four-blinks-script/

Chapter 6

# Endless Growth: Oraine Ramoo

Oraine Ramoo, MEd, is a women's counseling psychologist specializing in sexual and reproductive trauma in her home country of Trinidad and Tobago. During the past 16 years, she has worked exclusively with women, developing the Practical Applications in Trauma Healing Program (PATH) in 2010. This unique approach blends various trauma-processing modalities, somatic work, storytelling, mythology, and alternative therapies to support women through childhood sexual abuse and sexual assault.

As an EMDRIA-approved consultant, Oraine offers individualized guidance to consultees on enhancing their skills in EMDR processing, with an emphasis on conceptualization, strong resource utilization, and working with dissociation.

Oraine also works with flower essences and essential oils as a complementary medicine practitioner, often incorporating both into her counseling as a Bach Foundation registered practitioner and a National Association for Holistic Aromatherapy Level 1 aromatherapist. She is currently undertaking studies in mythology and logotherapy to add a deeper, unique layer to supporting her clients during and after trauma therapy.

## Which books have influenced your work as a therapist?

***Trauma and Beyond: The Mystery of Transformation* by Ursula Wirtz**

This book was written by a clinical and anthropological psychologist, and Jungian analyst. It reminds me that the counseling profession allows us to access the threads that connect with a client's soul fractures. People have grappled with suffering throughout history; symbols and mythic thinking play a role in the healing process. This is no easy task to undertake and requires deep trust in ourselves and our clients.

The modern therapist often gets caught up in training, modalities, insurance, online marketing, and more. In the process, they may forget the offering clients place before us with hopeful vulnerability, which may open space for something new, not simply restoring what was.

***Holy Listening: The Art of Spiritual Direction*** **by Margaret Guenther**

This book was written by an Episcopal priest, spiritual director, and former professor of ascetical theology at The General Theological Seminary in New York. Although this book is about spiritual direction, many excellent therapists also engage in similar practices in their work. Guenther calls it being a "midwife to the soul." It reminds me again of the sacredness of bearing witness to another's stories and the blessing of creating a space where healing can emerge—all while doing so with humility.

## How do you explain EMDR to clients?

I asked a graphic artist to design what I call the River Explanation. After sharing about the adaptive information processing (AIP) model, I further explain how feeder memories work using that illustration. The main river is the target, and the tributaries are the feeder memories that occurred earlier and may be confounding the current issue. Once we work on these memories, we eventually reach a place of calm: the Sea of Resolution.

*We eventually reach a place of calm: the Sea of Resolution.*

I always tell clients that we'll begin EMDR with a small, manageable memory first. This allows them to experience how the process works in a safe way before addressing more challenging material. While explanations and visuals are helpful, the best way to understand EMDR is to try it and experience it personally.

## What advice do you have for new EMDR therapists?

**Start identifying cases you can work with**. They do not need to be complex or even trauma related. We can use EMDR for anxiety, grief, depression, and much more. Keeping in mind the phases of EMDR, your treatment planning of identifying targets (phase 1) and especially resourcing (phase 2) are fertile places to get started.

**Seek out quality consultation early on.** The 10 hours mandated for basic training are good, but once that's out of the way, most therapists struggle with case conceptualization, remembering important cues, how to integrate EMDR into their practice, deciding which clients are a good fit, how to blend it with their other existing trainings, and how to troubleshoot issues. Early and excellent consultation can address all these concerns, build confidence, and prevent therapeutic drift.

**Network with EMDR practitioners.** Immerse yourself in EMDR communities and connect with like-minded individuals; there is so much to learn. You will need their training resources, book recommendations, cheering on, and self-care support. It can be overwhelming at first, but networking can help you parse what you need to focus on.

**Consider additional EMDR reading**. Honestly, more can also be overwhelming. But a basic text about EMDR is a great support just after basic training, when your brain is a bit muddled. Ask your consultant or network for recommendations, and select one or two that resonate with you.

**Join EMDRIA or the professional body of your country or choice.** It isn't mandatory, but the major benefits include access to its network, on-demand training, research, conference access, and resources. There are also opportunities to contribute by being on a committee, writing articles, teaching, and more.

## What did you intuitively know without formal training?

Clients can speak during processing! I've had sessions where clients speak during bilateral stimulation (BLS), even though I don't model it when explaining the process. I was not explicitly taught that clients should not do this.

However, there are times when I have not stopped them because it felt as if they needed to do so, and it appears to be beneficial to the client to share their experience in more detail as processing takes place. I also gain more information that can be applied appropriately at later junctures in our work.

Whenever I've encountered EMDR, whether in training videos or consultee videos, I've seen clients speaking during BLS only a couple of times. Yes, they can discuss what they are processing if it is beneficial to them and allows the trauma to move.

## What is one therapeutic approach that integrates well with EMDR?

Deep Brain Reorienting (DBR), developed by Frank Corrigan, is very effective. DBR works by tracking and processing the body's initial, instinctive physical reactions—known as "orienting tensions"—that occur just before a traumatic response fully develops. By focusing on these subtle, often unnoticed sensations in the brain stem, DBR allows the nervous system to safely reprocess the stored trauma at its source, leading to resolution and improved emotion regulation without requiring the person to relive the traumatic event.

When we begin DBR, one of the first things a client can experience is a release of the initial startle or shock that precedes a traumatic event. I usually facilitate this specific aspect of DBR just before phase 4, once the client has identified the target and subjective units of disturbance (SUD), but *not* the negative cognition. It is a very somatic technique. In subsequent sessions, the SUD on the target often drops significantly, and we then move forward with EMDR reprocessing.

## Which EMDR intervention have you found particularly effective?

Some clients have significantly benefited from early EMDR intervention (EEI), specifically the Recent Traumatic Episode Protocol (R-TEP) developed by Elan Shapiro and Brurit Laub. This training was timely for me. The very weekend I was being trained in the protocol, I received a call from a former client who shared that a family friend had just been the victim of an attempted armed robbery. Another friend who was present and licensed to carry a firearm shot the perpetrator directly in front of her; the bullet passed in front of her face. The perpetrator was killed.

I accepted the referral and scheduled her for that Monday. We spent two hours working intensively with R-TEP. I let her rest and integrate on Tuesday, and checked in on Wednesday. I was floored. She reported that she had slept well both nights; the acrid scent was gone from her nostrils, the sound of the shot had faded, and she felt much better.

Notably, if a client presents with the smell left behind after firing a gun in their nostrils or memories, eucalyptus essential oil can help neutralize the smell.

## Has a client's cultural background ever influenced your EMDR approach?

One of Trinidad and Tobago's most beautiful features is the blend of various cultures. We have descendants of India, Africa, France, Portugal, Venezuela, the UK, Syria, Lebanon, Grenada, China, Korea, and the indigenous Amerindian populations of the Caribs and Arawaks. They have sustained their religions, celebrations, foods, and mythologies.

I had a Muslim client, and we had to resource her nurturing, wise, and protective figures. She chose Allah for each, which I understood, but I felt that something was not quite robust about it. Years earlier, I had another Muslim client introduce me to the "99 Names of Allah," and I mentioned this. For reference, the 99 Names of Allah represent the 99 attributes of God, and each name is listed in Arabic.

The client then seemed to grasp what I had been attempting to do. She chose two names for each figure, totaling six resources. We had "The Avenger," "The Guide to the Right Path," "The All-Wise," and so forth. It worked beautifully. When she needed to bring in one of her figures, she would imagine the most fitting name of Allah's virtue in Arabic, and it would move the processing along.

## What is one mistake that turned into an opportunity for growth?

Before certification, I didn't fully understand which target to focus on after building the timeline. I thought it should be the worst experience, the most recent one, or the one that felt most challenging to the client. This led me to abandon a target and shift to material that appeared during phase 4, setting that up instead. It happened often, especially when I wasn't working on a single incident, and it wasted time.

During certification consults, I learned that working from the earliest target to the most recent yields "cleaner" results. The metaphor was that of a flowering plant: Start at the roots and move up the stem, clearing each issue so it doesn't become a feeder for later targets, which means less interference as we progress. That changed everything about how I conceptualize treatment and targets, and how I came up with the River Explanation.

> *Start at the roots and move up the stem, clearing each issue so it doesn't become a feeder for later targets.*

Sessions move faster, and I feel more efficient and organized. The client benefits from faster and improved healing outcomes by understanding how one or more experiences or events can compound others, causing complex mental and emotional responses.

## What EMDR success story caught you by surprise?

About three months after basic training, and while still completing my 10 hours, I received a referral for a woman who had lost her husband most tragically just a couple of weeks earlier. It was harrowing even to hear it. I was aware of Francine Shapiro's Recent Traumatic Event Protocol (RTE) and chose to apply it. It was challenging, as I was still getting accustomed to EMDR, let alone navigating this new-to-me protocol. I dove in. This was at the end of August.

By October, my client was singing the praises of EMDR to the high heavens. She spent long minutes mesmerized by how she felt, trying to process it. I, too, was trying to figure out how what felt like a chaotic series of sessions somehow worked so well. She is thriving and continues to refer people to me for EMDR. I had to speak with her once and explain that not every client is a candidate for EMDR. Her response was: "They need to be!" Since then, I have been trained in the R-TEP protocol and have been actively using it.

## References

Corrigan, F. M., & Christie-Sands, J. (2019). An innate brainstem self-other system involving orienting, affective responding, and polyvalent relational seeking: Some clinical implications for a "Deep Brain Reorienting" trauma psychotherapy approach. Medical Hypotheses, 136, 109502.

Guenther, M. (1992). Holy listening: The art of spiritual direction. Cowley Publications.

Shapiro, E., & Laub, B. (2008). Early EMDR intervention (EEI): A summary, a theoretical model, and the Recent Traumatic Episode Protocol (R-TEP). Journal of EMDR Practice and Research, 2(2), 79–96.

Shapiro, F. (2017). Eye movement desensitization and reprocessing (EMDR) therapy: Basic principles, protocols, and procedures (3rd ed.). Guilford Press.

Wirtz, U. (2020). Trauma and beyond: The mystery of transformation. Routledge.

# Chapter 7

# The Art of EMDR: Jocelyn Fitzgerald

Jocelyn Fitzgerald, LMFT, is an art therapist, an EMDRIA-approved consultant, and an author. With a passion for integrating creativity with trauma-focused therapy, she co-wrote *EMDR and the Creative Arts Therapies* and the children's book *Colorful Place: Mindful Story and Art for Kids*.

An accomplished speaker, Jocelyn has presented at national conferences and has been published in both popular and peer-reviewed publications, including *Psychotherapy Networker* magazine and scholarly journals in the fields of trauma and expressive therapies. She specializes in using art and EMDR to help people of all ages manage anxiety, process trauma, and build resilience. Based in Vancouver, Washington, Jocelyn also mentors clinicians on incorporating EMDR into their practice, emphasizing its transformative potential for healing and self-awareness.

## How do you explain EMDR to your clients?

I explain EMDR to clients by using an image I've created. I show them that EMDR is an eight-phase model and is different from traditional talk therapy. What makes it unique is the use of bilateral stimulation, which could be eye movements, tappers that create vibrations back and forth, or alternating sounds.

I explain that, after trauma, the amygdala—the brain's "firefighter"—activates, storing memories in ways that cause intense reactions, as if reliving the trauma. This is a normal evolutionary response: Our brains try to protect us. Even when safe, we can still react to non-threatening triggers.

EMDR helps by reactivating the traumatic memory while keeping clients within their window of tolerance. Bilateral stimulation helps the brain shift trauma from the amygdala to the frontal cortex. Although reprocessing doesn't erase the memory, the client stops reacting as intensely to it.

I emphasize EMDR's strong research support and its effectiveness for trauma. I offer clients resources, such as book and article recommendations, based on their preferences and interests.

## What advice do you have for new EMDR therapists?

Newly trained EMDR clinicians may be afraid of flooding their clients or worried about flashbacks, panic attacks, or the client feeling completely overwhelmed. This is an understandable response. Working with trauma is hard and can feel intimidating. But EMDR is safe and effective when done correctly. Here are tips for new EMDR therapists:

**Practice on yourself and with a partner.** I believe that experiencing EMDR as a client is key to understanding its power. In basic training, you get to practice on yourself and with a partner, but more practice is often needed to feel truly confident.

**Record your sessions and watch them.** Watching your recorded sessions, although awkward at first, helps build self-awareness. You'll see where you're confident and where you hesitate; this accelerates growth.

*Watching your recorded sessions, although awkward at first, helps build self-awareness.*

**Follow the protocol.** The EMDR protocol exists for a reason—it works. When in doubt, return to it. It provides a clear road map for what to do next, and sticking to it helps you stay grounded and focused during sessions.

**Get quality consultation.** Find a consultant with whom you feel comfortable working, or connect with other EMDR therapists who have more experience. Bring up the moments when you feel stuck or unsure. The EMDR community is supportive; you don't have to figure it out alone.

**Journal and make art about your own experiences.** Reflect on your personal EMDR work; write, meditate, or use creative expression. This deepens your understanding, enabling you to guide clients with empathy and clarity.

## What is one therapeutic approach that integrates really well with EMDR?

One key approach that I integrate with EMDR is the creative arts. I've used it since the very beginning. I still remember during basic training wishing each of the acronyms could come to life through images—something visual to help reflect what we're asking of clients during EMDR.

For example, I created an art piece that visually represents the subjective units of disturbance level (0 to 10) as calm ocean waters moving up to a giant tsunami wave. For the validity of cognition scale, which moves in the opposite direction, from 1 (completely false) to 7 (completely true), I created an image of a tiny seed growing into a sunflower in full bloom. For many clients, these numeric scales can feel overwhelming or confusing. But when they see the visuals, it clicks, and they understand the concept more intuitively.

I also incorporate art into phase 2, preparation, inviting clients to draw their safe state. Adding texture, meaning, and imagery enhances the experience. As they consider colors, shapes, and feelings while creating, the resource becomes more tangible and easier to access.

Recently, I've been incorporating AI art into this process, especially with clients who are fearful of or resistant to the traditional creative arts process. Clients have created their containers using AI-generated images, such as a box with the Batman symbol, a fierce mama bear guarding their memories, or a container at the bottom of the ocean surrounded by puffed-up puffer fish, ready to defend anything that tries to escape. Visuals help clients connect with their internal work on a deeper level, making it easier to remember and access resources between sessions.

*Visuals help clients connect with their internal work on a deeper level, making it easier to remember and access resources between sessions.*

Another favorite technique is the Inner Landscape Collage, whereby clients fill a body outline with collage materials that represent their internal feelings and sensations. I introduce weather metaphors (such as stormy, foggy, or sunny) to help clients translate sensations and emotions into visual, symbolic language.

One client I'd worked with for several years was preparing to leave for college. Matias often described strange sensations in his body and said he didn't feel stable. We did EMDR around a challenging situation in his relationship and then decided to use art to map his physical sensations.

Matias randomly selected images and glued them to his body outline. When he finished, we stepped back to look at the patterns he'd created. At the bottom of the outline, he had glued icicles. Matias pointed to them and said, "These icicles represent my cold feet. I'm not feeling ready to leave for college—I'm terrified. I haven't told my parents this, but I don't want to go. I feel pushed into a major that doesn't align with who I am, and I don't even know what I want to do yet."

This simple collage gave him clear imagery to explore his fears. Through creativity, he clarified his experience. We planned how Matias would address his fears with his parents. In the next session, we used EMDR's future template to process his fears and rehearse the conversation. We built a supportive plan aligned with his vision for the future.

Art complements EMDR by visually expressing internal work, helping clients understand themselves, track progress, and carry healing beyond the therapy room. Integrating art with EMDR opens doors for clients, especially those who struggle to find words to express what they're feeling. It doesn't have to be perfect or pretty—it just has to be expressive and real. When clients create something visual to represent their healing, it becomes a reminder of their strength, progress, and the work they're doing, even long after the session ends.

> *Integrating art with EMDR opens doors for clients, especially those who struggle to find words to express what they're feeling.*

## Which EMDR intervention have you found particularly effective?

I created an exercise while working with Ethiopian refugee teens. What struck me most was how disconnected many of them were from their bodies. Initially, it felt like many images were floating heads, with very little awareness of the body or sensation. Before we could begin EMDR, it became clear that we first needed to help them reconnect with their whole selves.

One powerful way to do this is with art. Using creative techniques, we can gently explore and map what we're feeling inside our bodies. This exercise is one I often return to with clients, and I've found it both impactful and deeply grounding.

### Art- and Body-Based Transformation Exercise

This exercise is designed for use during phase 2 of EMDR, preparation. It helps clients develop awareness of how emotions and sensations are held in the body and supports grounding, resourcing, and readiness for later phases of trauma processing.

**When to Introduce**

Introduce this exercise early in phase 2, after clients have been oriented to the EMDR process. It's helpful for clients who struggle with body awareness, feel disconnected from their emotions, or need to build additional stability before moving into reprocessing.

**How to Introduce**

Invite the client to choose a mild or moderately stressful memory (SUD level 1 to 4). Explain the purpose of creating a body map: to gently notice where and how the body holds feelings, using colors and shapes. Encourage them to approach the exercise with curiosity and self-compassion, not judgment. Remind them that this is a resourcing tool, not a reprocessing tool, designed to build connection and capacity in the present moment. Consider incorporating bilateral tapping after each art process to deepen integration and strengthen the mind-body connection.

Here's how I explain it:

*Trauma can create a disconnect between the mind and body, leaving us feeling detached from emotions and physical sensations. This exercise invites you to gently reconnect with your body through creative expression, noticing where stress, sadness, or fear might be stored.*

*Using colors, lines, and shapes, you'll create a "body map" to represent how your body holds difficult experiences. This practice can help you become more present, build awareness, and begin transforming old patterns into healing pathways.*

**Materials Needed**

- Colored pens or pencils
- A pen for writing
- The Map It Out worksheet

**Step-by-Step Instructions**

1. Center yourself. Before beginning, take a few slow breaths and check in with your body. Notice where you feel grounded and where you feel tension.

2. Identify a stressful memory. Think of a mildly stressful experience from your past. Using a 0 to 10 scale, where 0 is no stress and 10 is the most stress you could imagine, pick a memory that's a 3 or 4. Write the number at the bottom of the paper in the square. Next, describe the experience in a few words: What happened? When and where did it occur?

3. Fill in the Map It Out worksheet. Using colors and shapes, show where you feel the sensations connected to this memory. Let them express your internal experience. For example:

- Swirls in the stomach = nervousness
- Red rings around the throat = sadness
- Blue tears in the eyes = grief

4. Identify your negative belief. What did you believe about yourself in that moment? Write it down below your body map, for example, "I'm not good enough," "I'm not safe," or "I can't handle this."

5. Rate the intensity. On a 0 to 10 scale, how intense does this memory feel right now?

6. Close your eyes and scan your body. Notice where you feel tension or discomfort. Use your fingers to gently tap one side of your art paper with your left hand, then your right, back and forth for about one minute.

7. Write a new, positive belief you'd like to hold, for example, "I'm strong," "I'm capable," or "I'm safe now." Draw over your original body map using new colors and shapes, letting the new belief flow into your artwork.

8. Once again, gently tap back and forth on your paper, reinforcing the new positive belief with bilateral stimulation.

## What creative modifications have you made to EMDR to address specific populations or presenting issues?

I use the creative arts in EMDR in many ways. For example, when introducing resourcing and helping clients access a safe state, we often move beyond talking. I invite clients to create a collage using images that represent safety for them, such as a cozy blanket, a loyal dog, or someone holding a warm cup of tea. These images help stimulate a felt sense of safety in the body, even if just for a brief moment, and can strengthen the neural pathways that connect feeling safe to physical sensation.

*I invite clients to create a collage using images that represent safety for them*

One client, a nurse with a long history of abuse from both a narcissistic father and an ex-husband, had experienced extensive trauma that manifested physically through chronic pain, multiple surgeries, and an autoimmune disorder. In our work together, Hana began mapping the areas of her body where she felt pain using colors, lines, and shapes.

She described her chest as housing a broken heart, shattered and trembling, with fire radiating from her stomach. Hana's feet, which had been operated on multiple times, felt fragmented and fragile, expressed through jagged lines. From her hands emerged what she called the draining of all her "hopes and dreams."

As we processed these sensations through EMDR, Hana explored the deep sense of betrayal she felt toward her body. Once the EMDR work was complete, I invited her to lay tracing paper over the original image of her body map and consider: *What parts of your body now feel healing or strong?*

In this next layer, Hana transformed the fire and broken heart into symbolic dumbbell weights, representing her inner strength and the ways she had turned her trauma into advocacy for her students. She was attuned to the needs of children who had experienced trauma, often sensing when they were in distress and stepping in as a fierce protector.

Hana also loved mythology, and in a powerful reframe, chose to draw wings coming out of her feet, inspired by Hermes, the winged Greek god. She said these wings symbolized the gratitude she felt toward her medical team and her ability to rise again and move forward, despite surgeries and setbacks.

At the end of the session, she looked at her transformed body map and said, "Because of my pain, I can now see my strengths. Without the pain I experienced in the past, I wouldn't be the person I am today."

> *Because of my pain, I can now see my strengths.*

This story highlights the power of combining EMDR with creative expression. When we provide clients with opportunities to visualize, externalize, and transform their internal experiences through art, we access something deeply healing and profoundly empowering.

## What self-care practices do you engage in regularly?

One of my favorite self-care practices is seeing a great trauma therapist. I always say, "Trauma therapists are only as good as the trauma therapists they see." Doing deep, intense work requires a strong understanding of yourself, especially knowing where you might get triggered, so you can support clients without carrying their pain into your own life.

> *Trauma therapists are only as good*
> *as the trauma therapists they see.*

I also incorporate other forms of self-care that keep me grounded. I get regular massages and bodywork, which help release stress and reconnect me to my body. My morning ritual is another cornerstone. Each day starts with making tea and spending time doing art while listening to music, meditating, or reciting a poem. I also take a few moments to journal, set an intention, and write down something I'm grateful for.

Exercise is a big part of how I care for my mental health. It's as essential for my mind as it is for my body. As someone prone to anxiety, a good cardio workout helps reset my nervous system and keeps me grounded after tough sessions.

For me, learning is a form of self-care. I constantly read, sign up for trainings, and dive into creative or business-focused courses. When I began this work, I didn't realize how much growth and learning would be involved, but it has become one of my favorite aspects of the job. Staying curious and inspired keeps me feeling fresh and excited to show up for my clients and my practice.

## References

Davis, E., et. al, (2022). EMDR and the Creative Arts Therapies. Routledge.

Fitzgerald, J. (2019). Colorful place: Mindful story and art for kids. Independently published.

Fitzgerald, J. (2023). AI and therapy: Creativity, ethics, and the future of the therapeutic relationship. Psychotherapy Networker. https://www.psychotherapynetworker.org

Shapiro, F. (2001). Eye movement desensitization and reprocessing: Basic principles, protocols, and procedures (2nd ed.). Guilford Press.

Shapiro, F. (2018). Eye movement desensitization and reprocessing (EMDR) therapy: Basic principles, protocols, and procedures (3rd ed.). Guilford Press.

Shapiro, F., Kaslow, F. W., & Maxfield, L. (2007). Handbook of EMDR and family therapy processes. John Wiley & Sons.

# Chapter 8

# The Joining of Jung and Shapiro: Andrew Dobo

For Andrew Dobo, PsyD, a journey in psychology began in 1976 while he was an undergraduate studying music composition in Chicago. The city, a haven for musicians in the 1970s, was full of bookstores and record stores. One day, he came across *Modern Man in Search of His Soul* by Carl G. Jung. This discovery marked the beginning of an inward exploration that transformed his path.

Andrew was introduced to EMDR in 1998 at Florida Tech during his doctoral training. One day, a local therapist presented at his school. She waved her hand in front of a student volunteer's eyes and reduced his anxiety about an issue in approximately 15 minutes. A few weeks later, Andrew followed up and confirmed the student was still free of anxiety about the issue.

Fortunately, one of Andrew's professors had been trained in EMDR by Francine Shapiro in the early 1990s, when EMDR was in its infancy. After 25 years and thousands of EMDR sessions, Andrew now has the privilege of training therapists.

He is the author of three books: *Unburdening Souls at the Speed of Thought: Psychology, Christianity, and the Transforming Power of EMDR*; *The Hero's Journey: Integrating EMDR Therapy and Jungian Psychology*; and *Transformational EMDR: The Manual—Shapiro's Aspiration for EMDR Beyond the Disease Model.*

## Which books have influenced your work as a therapist?

***Healing and Wholeness* by John A. Sanford**

This book by a Jungian analyst and Episcopal minister is a masterpiece that explains how the psyche functions in our lives. I've read this book at least 20 times since I first picked it up in 1977; even now, I still find things I didn't remember or didn't fully understand. More than any other, this book helped me understand, on a deep level, what happens during EMDR therapy.

People often forget that Francine Shapiro identified EMDR as a psychoanalytic process. She did so in 1990, when she changed the name from "EMD"—where she believed the process desensitized an image—to "EMDR" to reflect the free association component of psychoanalytic therapy. That approach evolved into instructing the therapist not to interfere and instead to allow whatever emerges to unfold naturally. Jung and Freud both employed this style—the therapist as a "blank slate." Therapists are rarely trained in the language of the unconscious. Sanford's book is a great place to start learning and understanding the language that shows up in EMDR therapy.

***Subtract: The Untapped Science of Less* by Leidy Klotz**

This book warns about adding elements to a system that actually make it weaker. Adding to EMDR's standard protocol without justification has caused immense harm by weakening its effectiveness. This book tells us that, in reality, doing the opposite of adding—subtracting—often makes a system more powerful, efficient, and effective. It reminds us that humans are hardwired to add things in the name of improvement, but this often does more harm than good. Shapiro warned of this very problem in her keynote at EMDRIA in 2003.

This problem is far worse today, to the point that EMDR is often unrecognizable. Shapiro's complaint about tampering with the model dates back to 2003, and it's even more relevant now. She said in her keynote address, "We have had an upsurge in clients calling the institute over the past year, saying, 'I'm really confused. I've been doing EMDR for weeks or months. I love my clinician—we have a great rapport and I feel great at the end of every session. But when I go home, my issues are still there. I'm just not getting any better. I read this book, and it doesn't sound like what they're doing is EMDR.'"

***The Genius Myth* by Michael Meade**

This is an incredible book that explains how to access our inner genius—and that of our clients. That access comes by getting into a state of "flow." While Meade doesn't explicitly use the term "flow," he describes everything involved in reaching it. And you can't access your inner genius unless you're in flow.

> *You can't access your inner genius unless you're in flow.*

## How do you explain EMDR to your clients?

I approach each person differently and use a perspective they can relate to. To explain EMDR, I often use the REM Theory, which highlights elements that distinguish EMDR from other therapies. My explanation might go something like this:

*EMDR stands for "eye movement desensitization and reprocessing." It has its beginnings in 1987, when a doctoral student noticed that moving her eyes rapidly back and forth while thinking about a distressing memory reduced its emotional intensity. After experimenting with the phenomenon, she developed a standardized therapeutic protocol and formally established EMDR therapy.*

*It is linked to rapid eye movement (REM) sleep, because some scientists believe that EMDR uses the same mechanism as REM sleep; something similar happens when information is being processed.*

*REM sleep helps process daily events by sorting and reducing unnecessary emotions in our memories. If something upsetting happens, like almost getting in an accident, REM helps settle those feelings by the next day. It lets us remember the event without reliving the strong emotions.*

*Tomorrow, if you tell someone what happened, you won't feel the experience all over again. You'll just think of it as something that happened—not much different from what you bought at the grocery store yesterday. It becomes just something that happened.*

*REM processes the emotional and sensory aspects of memories, leaving behind only what's necessary to remember. EMDR appears to do something similar. Traumatic events—or even everyday stress—can disrupt REM. REM sleep can't always handle overwhelming experiences, and as a result, the information doesn't move to where it's supposed to go in the brain. That leaves parts of the memory unprocessed and able to influence our mood, reactions, and life.*

*EMDR acts like an enhanced REM, helping process memories that REM can't handle. It reduces a memory's emotional impact, leaving a more neutral experience.*

*EMDR acts like an enhanced REM, helping process memories that REM can't handle.*

## What is your approach to addressing ambivalence or hesitation when introducing EMDR to clients?

I ask the client something like, "Are you ever troubled by this memory during the day or night?" Or "Does the memory ever intrude while you're driving or while you're trying to fall asleep?" Usually, they say, "Of course—you know it does."

I then tell them, "All I'm asking you to do with EMDR is to allow that to happen here with me, safely, while you hold these tappers and wear these headphones. I'm not asking you to do anything that doesn't already happen to you. The only difference is, if you do it here with me, it won't trouble you again."

This is a powerful way to break through ambivalence; yet some people still resist.

## What advice do you have for new EMDR therapists?

**Get certified!** The reason is simple: You don't know what you don't know. Taking a course that teaches integrating another model into EMDR shouldn't happen until you've developed a deep understanding of what's really going on in EMDR. Why? Because without that understanding, when a problem arises, you'll say, "EMDR isn't working," and then use an intervention that doesn't help either. It's not that EMDR isn't working; it's that you're missing 80 percent of what's happening with the client and the EMDR process. Certification is a necessary and thoughtful next step.

> *It's not that EMDR isn't working; it's that you're missing 80 percent of what's happening with the client and the EMDR process.*

**Seek out someone who knows volumes more than you**. Get certified with someone who, if possible, has written a book. Don't be afraid to ask high-profile people. Find a consultant who's willing to watch videos of your sessions. Try not to work with someone who's only been doing EMDR a year or two longer than you. Look for someone with 10 to 20 years of experience.

**Interview the consultant.** You shouldn't feel intimidated by your consultant. If they make you feel small instead of like they're your biggest fan, move on. Any teacher or supervisor worth their salt knows you get the best out of people by making them feel safe.

Make sure they have a sense of humor and that they're passionate about EMDR—not just as an academic practice, but as an art.

**Secure a consultant who's creative, passionate, and able to laugh at themselves.** In *The Genius Myth*, Meade talks about the archetype of the sacred king versus the poisonous king. You might think of Volodymyr Zelenskyy as the sacred king and Vladimir Putin as the poisonous one. Supervisors and consultants fall into similar archetypal power roles. Find one who is creative, passionate, and able to laugh at themselves.

**Avoid collecting certifications.** Don't sign up for certifications that offer four hours of credit on a Saturday afternoon. You won't be any better at EMDR on Sunday than you were on Friday. Collecting certifications as fast as possible goes against the spirit of EMDRIA certification—but people do it. People who are driven by the negative cognition "I'm not good enough" tend to do it. The more letters you've got after your name, the more urgently you need EMDR to help neutralize that belief—and the sooner you'll be brave enough to show your work to someone skilled. Find someone to watch recorded videos with you; you'll get very good, very fast.

## What did you intuitively know that wasn't addressed in a training?

There was little to no focus on what abreactions can be like—or what to do when one happens. Shapiro's 2003 keynote emphasized—and warned—that a therapist's fear can impede the EMDR process, particularly when they're afraid of a client's intense emotions.

I knew a client would have to reexperience the event to some degree. I was never afraid of people being on the floor wailing, because Shapiro normalized that for me. Her keynote emphasized the need for EMDR therapists to develop a high tolerance for affect—and I did. I listened to that speech off and on for more than a year, until I could practically recite it.

I also intuitively knew that dreams are an essential part of any meaningful therapeutic process. I had decades of experience with dreams and found them personally essential. I welcomed it when EMDR clients brought their dreams into session. I noticed that many clients had similar dream themes, likely because they were going through the same therapeutic process. EMDR accelerates movement in the psyche, and that's clearly reflected in dreams.

> *Dreams are an essential part of any meaningful therapeutic process.*

There are distinct stages clients move through, and their dreams tend to reflect those stages. The six stages are:

- Avoidance
- Surrender
- Dismantling the old way
- Chaos, confusion, and loss of identity
- Rebirth: accepting the new way
- Assimilating the new way

Each stage brings its own dream themes. Yet, most EMDR trainings don't discuss dreams at all. Carl Rogers concluded that clients improve not because of what the therapist says, or because of the theory being used; they improve because of their own internal experiences. EMDR creates those internal experiences—just like dreams do. Sadly, dreams aren't seen as the powerfully transformational internal experiences they truly are within the EMDR ecosystem.

## What is one therapeutic approach that integrates really well with EMDR?

A therapeutic approach that integrates really well with EMDR is the Jungian model—or any psychoanalytic model, really. That said, I prefer not to use the word "integrate." Psychoanalytic models aren't something you add into EMDR; they're already an integral part of it. EMDR is a psychoanalytic therapy, but few EMDR therapists are trained in the process or the language.

Shapiro recommends the psychoanalytic method, and the language of the psyche naturally emerges in the session. It's up to the therapist to recognize it and use it to enhance generalization, which reduces the time spent in phase 4. The language of the unconscious is easy to explain, and with a little practice, it becomes easy to recognize, understand, and work with.

The psychoanalytic language is unremarkable on the surface. But the phrases that come from this part of the psyche are often highly generalizable—and therefore, deeply healing. These phrases are applicable in various contexts. Take the phrase, "I've got to get out of here." That could apply to someone who's afraid of elevators or airplanes. But it could just as easily apply if your big brother locked you in a closet at age five, or if your violent husband locked you in a bathroom before beating you. That one seemingly simple phrase can be the connective tissue linking dozens of memories.

You want to develop an ear for this. Using these kinds of phrases can shorten the time in phase 4 and enhance generalization to memories across the lifespan—sometimes far from the original target. Recognizing psychoanalytic language is where the real power of EMDR lies. That's why watching recordings is so important. When I watch tape with a consultee, I can point out these phrases—the ones that are easy to overlook.

> *Recognizing psychoanalytic language*
> *is where the real power of EMDR lies.*

There's a lot of discussion about somatization, such as asking, "Where do you feel it in your body?" I never ask that question. It breaks the flow instantly. When a client reports a body sensation, psychoanalytic models suggest three possible meanings. Let's say the client says, "My neck is starting to hurt."

1. It could be a traumatic reenactment. Maybe the client was strangled or abused, and that's the source of the pain. I might say, "Go with that.... Allow yourself to feel that neck pain."

2. The pain could be a message from the unconscious. I might use an interweave, respecting the message by asking, "Is anyone a pain in your neck right now?" Often, someone comes to mind, and we go with that. The pain usually resolves. Every body part has a metaphor. The unconscious uses metaphors to communicate.

1. It could connect to a source memory through a somatic bridge or floatback.

> You discover this by using the somatic floatback technique. The somatic bridge was developed by John and Helen Watkins, hypnotherapists who had a deep understanding of the unconscious mind. William Zangwill wasn't trained in hypnosis, but he adapted the floatback for the EMDR community.

These examples are just the tip of the iceberg. Learning the language of the psyche is essential. Once you understand it, you may find that other integrations actually dilute the power of EMDR.

## What role does attachment theory play in your EMDR practice?

None. If someone has an unhealthy attachment, they're usually driven by the cognition: "I don't matter." I address the attachment by helping shift the "I don't matter" cognition to "I do matter." This is not just any cognition. It's a transformative shift that can cause cataclysmic change for the client.

If someone has an unhealthy attachment, what caused it? It's usually because their caregiver didn't provide what was needed. What does that mean? It means the client wasn't significant enough. They didn't matter. Something else was more important.

The process of healing through EMDR can be treacherous and, at the same time, exuberantly transformative. I keep things very simple. I don't frame it through attachment theory—I frame it through cognition.

## What EMDR success story caught you by surprise?

Jung's concept of synchronicity refers to a meaningful coincidence—an acausal event that occurs when something from the inner world of imagination breaks through into our three-dimensional outer world. If you don't have a relationship with your inner self, synchronistic events often go unnoticed. But sometimes the inner world forces its hand, as you'll see in the following story.

## The Case of the Barking Dog

The client was a 55-year-old male with a history of trauma. Kristof's emotionally abusive mother told him from a young age that he was unwanted, a mistake, and that she had wanted to kill herself after his birth. The plan was to address the many abusive events from childhood—until the barking dog entered the story.

Kristof arrived at session visibly agitated by his wife's dog—a dog he's very fond of. He immediately began ranting about the dog's behavior that morning.

"I never heard the dog bark like that before. I couldn't get him to stop. It was barking and barking. No matter what I did, it wouldn't stop. It was out of control. There was no reason for it—nothing going on outside—but he wouldn't stop. It was like he was possessed. He never does that. I never saw him act like that before. I had to get out of there. I told my wife, 'I've got to get out of here. I'm going to Starbucks to get a coffee and go see Dobo.'"

On the surface, the barking dog seemed like a mere annoyance, and the plan was to focus on the client's hateful mother. But if we see the barking dog through the lens of *the unconscious is an ally*, and if we treat every word the client says as potentially meaningful—even the nonsense—hidden doors start to open.

That barking dog revealed avoided material. Jung would call this "the shadow." Shapiro might describe it as "implicit memory fragments becoming explicit." By receiving—rather than *knowing*—a channel to hidden material was opened and processed. The barking dog was a synchronistic event according to Jung—the inner world intruding on the outer world—which is helpful in the therapy process.

> *By receiving—rather than knowing—a channel to hidden material was opened and processed.*

During reprocessing, the phrase "I've got to get out of here" linked to three separate situations where Kristof's life had been in danger—all stories he hadn't told me. The dog's barking made Kristof feel out of control, which triggered the phrase. That phrase was the key that connected to hidden traumas.

That's the essence of working from a psychoanalytic perspective. Trust that what you need will show up—you just have to recognize it. The barking dog could have been dismissed, and I could have gone back to the plan, focusing on the abusive mother. But psychoanalytic thinking finds meaning where others do not.

## References

Shapiro, F. (2003, September 18–21). The adaptive information processing model and case conceptualization [Keynote address]. EMDRIA Conference, Denver, Colorado.

# Chapter 9

# The Soul of EMDR: Alexandra Dent

The journey of Alexandra Dent, MPhil, DClinPsych, centers on seeking, embracing, and living her own spiritual and authentic truth, overcoming fear and prejudice along the way. It took many years, along with many personal challenges and traumas, for her to realize that the answer lay within her heart.

Part of Alexandra's journey involved training as a clinical psychologist, initially working within England's National Health Service (NHS) for Child and Adolescent Mental Health Services (CAMHS). In 2012, she began working independently with individuals across the age span, integrating spirituality more fully into her work.

Alexandra trained in EMDR in 2009 and became an EMDR Europe–accredited consultant in 2016, followed by a training facilitator designation two years later. She chaired the UK EMDR Child and Adolescent Committee for four years and has served as chair of the EMDR Association UK's Spirituality Specialist Interest Group since 2019. Alexandra is the author of *Using Spirituality in EMDR Therapy: The Heart-Led Approach*.

## What advice do you have for new EMDR therapists?

**Start using EMDR right away.** Do so as soon as you can after attending the course. If you don't use it, you are likely to lose it.

**Build your confidence.** If you have complex clients, consider finding simpler cases, perhaps through colleagues or friends of friends to build up your confidence in using the standard protocol.

**Engage EMDR peers.** Stay connected with other EMDR therapists, especially those you trained with, so you can practice together and encourage each other.

**Find an EMDR consultant early on.** Doing so can boost your motivation and help you apply EMDR to client cases, even in the history taking, formulation, and preparation phases.

**Return to the standard protocol.** There are many—perhaps too many—EMDR "protocols." All together, they can feel overwhelming when you're starting out. But remember, the standard protocol is still the core model. It works well in most cases without needing adjustment.

**Use adaptations wisely.** If you work with children, ensure that you attend an accredited child and adolescent EMDR training to adapt the standard protocol developmentally. Adaptations, like those for pain or addiction, should only be used when clinically justified.

**Avoid getting ahead of yourself.** Don't jump into too many advanced trainings before you've mastered the standard protocol. Once you've got that foundation, then seek further training—especially in dissociation, parts work, and attachment theory. One of my consultees attended numerous additional trainings but hadn't practiced the standard protocol. It was her way of managing her "I'm not good enough" part. In consultation, she presented cases where her clients were clearly dissociating, but she couldn't see it. Though eager to advance, skipping the basics meant it took her years to become accredited.

**Know and respect your limits.** You don't have to work with every type of client.

**Use a case formulation approach.** When building a treatment plan, remember that you don't have to process all of a client's traumas, even if they sound horrific to you. Select targets that are linked to their therapy goals and are likely to improve their current level of functioning, using a case formulation approach as recommended by Andrew Leeds.

*When building a treatment plan, remember that you don't have to process all of a client's traumas, even if they sound horrific to you.*

**Develop strong clinical skills.** EMDR is not just a technique or a tool. Some therapists criticize EMDR for not focusing enough on the therapeutic relationship or attachment in the basic training. However, EMDR assumes that you already have strong clinical skills. You'll need to learn to integrate those with the method. For some, this will come naturally, and for others it will take time.

## What did you intuitively know that wasn't addressed in a training?

Using my intuition.

I would never describe myself as an academic, and being dyslexic with an ADHD-style brain has meant that working memory has always been a challenge. I've never been able to hold facts and information the way some others seem to. While this has felt like a disadvantage in some areas of life, it's also allowed me to work intuitively and energetically with clients—which I've written about elsewhere.

I've had to learn how to recognize, trust, and develop these skills, as they were never taught to me and often contradicted the very cognitive world I grew up in. These "intuitive knowings" include clairvoyance (seeing), claircognizance (knowing), clairsentience (feeling), and clairaudience (hearing), and they guide me in both therapy and life. Self-care and ongoing personal healing are essential for these intuitive skills to deepen.

I utilize these skills throughout all phases of EMDR, from taking a client's history to formulating a treatment plan and identifying the resources that may be needed during preparation. During assessment, I often intuitively sense what the client's negative and positive cognitions will be—sometimes even before they say them.

During desensitization, I sometimes know what the client will say or feel before they speak it aloud. I'm often guided toward the right interweave, or how long to keep the bilateral stimulation (BLS) running. My intuition helps me know when to close a session, even if incomplete, and how to follow up with care and clarity. This energetic and intuitive guidance continues through all phases and acts as an internal compass, letting me know we're on track.

> *This energetic and intuitive guidance acts as an internal compass, letting me know we're on track.*

Of course, there are times when something interferes with that intuitive channel. When that happens, I explore whether it's my own material or parts getting in the way, or whether the client may be consciously or unconsciously blocking the connection on an energetic or spiritual level. I have a strong "intuitive alarm" that warns me when something doesn't feel right in a session. And the rare occasions when I've ignored it, it usually leads to a powerful lesson I need to learn—and integrate.

## What is one therapeutic approach that integrates really well with EMDR?

One of the main approaches I find especially compatible with EMDR is parts work. There are many forms of parts work, including ego state therapy, Internal Family Systems (IFS), Gestalt therapy, and dialectical behavior therapy (DBT), each with its own unique strengths. I believe it's about finding the approach that best fits your clinical style, rather than deciding one is better than another.

I trained in ego state work with EMDR in 2013, and it's been invaluable when working with complex dissociative presentations, especially during preparation. These days, my approach is best described as a blend of ego state strategies and IFS techniques.

If a client has experienced complex trauma and early attachment wounds, you can be sure they've learned to dissociate as a survival strategy. Most of us dissociate from time to time, but the extent to which clients rely on this strategy can vary widely. I strongly believe in conducting a comprehensive history early on—often alongside resource and stabilization work—to create a solid case formulation and treatment plan. My formulations are grounded in attachment and trauma theory and, where possible, informed by spiritual or energetic understanding. By this point, I typically have a clear sense of the client's dissociative patterns.

> *If a client has experienced complex trauma and early attachment wounds, you can be sure they've learned to dissociate.*

Protective parts may appear at any point in the therapy process. In some cases, it helps to begin parts work during the history taking and preparation phases, approaching the protective role of each part with compassionate curiosity to understand and support it. This approach helps validate the part's efforts, strengthens the therapeutic relationship, and often helps gain permission to access underlying trauma.

However, parts don't always emerge until phases 3 and 4, when they may block processing. If you've already introduced parts work, it can often be integrated into processing through interweaves or supportive dialogue. If not, consider pausing processing, returning to preparation, and doing the necessary parts work until the system feels safe and ready to continue.

## Which EMDR intervention have you found particularly effective?

I am passionate about bridging the gap between spirituality and science. Over the past 30 years, some EMDR therapists have recognized the relevance of a spiritual component in EMDR.

The heart has been a source of fascination in both Eastern and Western traditions for thousands of years. In the fourth century BCE, Aristotle recognized its importance, describing the heart as "The seat of the soul and the control of voluntary movement—in fact, of all nervous functions in general—are to be sought in the heart. The brain is an organ of minor importance."

Recent research suggests the heart is one of the most significant organs in the human body: It has its own nervous system, intuitive functions, and electromagnetic field.

Based on my clinical and personal journey, I developed Heart-Led Psychotherapy (HLP) as part of a broader biopsychosociospiritual approach to treating trauma and psychological distress. HLP offers two models—the Heart-Led model and the Heart-and-Soul-Led model—to guide therapists and clients in adopting a more authentic, heart-centered path to healing at a deeper, transpersonal level.

HLP works on the premise that each person is on a unique journey meant to explore and embody core life lessons such as empowerment, love, and forgiveness. When trauma or attachment injury occurs, it can create energetic and psychological blocks that may manifest as core negative beliefs such as, "I'm not good enough," "I'm unlovable," or "I'm bad." In HLP, the ego refers to overthinking, overanalysis, and self-image—mechanisms that keep clients stuck in cycles of powerlessness, fear, and self-victimization.

In HLP-informed EMDR, a comprehensive history helps identify a client's challenges, traumas, attachment wounds, and repeating life patterns. The next stage involves teaching mindfulness strategies, so that clients become observers of their own experience and begin to recognize emerging life lessons. Clients are also guided in building a relationship with their heart using meditation, imagery, and reflective practices. As the observers using these techniques, clients learn to make new choices that are heart-led, rather than ego-led, which are more in keeping with their true authentic selves.

> *Clients learn to make new choices that are heart-led, rather than ego-led, which are more in keeping with their true authentic selves.*

HLP can be used with anyone, regardless of their spiritual beliefs; it integrates easily with EMDR, facilitating transformational, multidimensional healing. Suggestions for integrating a spiritual- and heart-led approach into each EMDR phase include:

**Phase 1, history taking**

- Complete a detailed life history to identify traumas, blocks, and patterns.
- Ask clients, with compassionate curiosity, about their spiritual beliefs.
- Note any spiritual practices or resources they already use (for example, meditation, prayer, time in nature, creative expression).

**Phase 2, preparation**

- Install spiritual figures.
- Create a peaceful or spiritually meaningful place.
- Teach the container exercise, possibly integrating a spiritual element.
- Introduce formal and informal mindfulness strategies.
- Teach the HLP model and how to apply it in daily life.
- Integrate spiritual concepts into Resource Development and Installation (RDI).
- Teach meditative techniques such as light stream meditation, mindful breathing, heart meditations, and heart coherence.
- Use heart-based or spiritual affirmations.

**Phases 3 to 8, assessment through reevaluation**

- Identify whether negative and positive cognitions have a spiritual dimension. For example:
  - NC: “I am tainted.” → PC: “I have a heart full of love.”
  - NC: “I am powerless.” → PC: “I am divinely supported.”
  - NC: “I cannot trust myself.” → PC: “I am learning to trust in my heart/soul.”
- If the client becomes stuck, guide them to place attention on their heart. Use interweaves such as:
  - “What guidance is your heart offering right now?”

– "What might this experience be here to teach you?" (If you have taught them the HLP model.)

– "Can you send healing love and light from your heart to someone else, perhaps across generations or time?"

– Connect with spiritual resources.

– Use the two-handed interweave to explore and separate conflicting messages from the heart and ego.

For an incomplete session, ask what aspects of the work felt most meaningful. Identify a heart-led positive statement to install, such as: "I am learning to listen to my heart's guidance." Install heart-led positive cognitions at the end of a complete session.

Finally, incorporate heart-led and spiritual techniques into the three-pronged EMDR approach. This includes helping clients prepare for future challenges by making heart-led choices that align with their authenticity.

## What role does attachment theory play in your EMDR practice?

I believe that having a strong understanding of attachment theory is essential for EMDR clinicians, especially when working with more complex cases. Working with young people in CAMHS early in my clinical career provided me with a solid foundation in recognizing early attachment patterns and working within family systems.

I trained in dyadic developmental psychotherapy (DDP) earlier on in my career. I saw how beautifully DDP and EMDR can complement one another to provide a comprehensive, attachment- and trauma-informed treatment package.

The complexity of client presentations seems to have increased dramatically over the past five to 10 years. In my view, it's impossible to work effectively with complex clients without understanding their attachment histories. I'm still surprised to hear clinicians working with trauma who haven't explored early attachment as part of history taking. How can you work safely without knowing what inner attachment wounds a client may be carrying? These wounds significantly impact the therapeutic relationship and a client's ability to self-soothe and connect.

> *It's impossible to work effectively with complex clients without understanding their attachment histories.*

Clients with these wounds often learned to dissociate from their bodies, emotions, and sensations as a survival strategy. Without proper preparation, they're more likely to dissociate during processing.

I begin with a comprehensive history, which may take several sessions. However, if a client is especially fragile or dysregulated due to early attachment trauma, I prioritize stabilization, psychoeducation, mindfulness, and resource building first. This helps expand the client's window of tolerance before gathering more details.

When I do gather history, I avoid asking for in-depth trauma details too soon. Doing so can be triggering and unnecessary. Sometimes, I can tell that something significant has happened simply by observing a client's emotional response during a session, and I make a note of it. I aim to keep clients within their window of tolerance and adjust my approach accordingly. Babette Rothschild speaks to this beautifully in her book *The Body Remembers: The Psychophysiology of Trauma and Trauma Treatment*.

One tool I find invaluable is the genogram. It's a powerful way to explore family systems, uncover intergenerational trauma, and ask about medical and psychological patterns across generations, including of parents, siblings, children, grandparents, even cousins.

From an attachment lens, I also ask clients who made them feel safe, loved, or nurtured, and for examples. I explore whether the client experienced emotionally, cognitively, physically, or spiritually supportive caregiving, especially in the critical early years, or whether they were left to manage painful emotions on their own. That alone gives me a good sense of whether dissociation likely developed early as a coping strategy. These dissociative tendencies are likely to impact subsequent relationships at school and work, and in personal life and the therapy room.

Once I've created an attachment- and trauma-informed formulation, I often begin with parts work and attachment-based strategies, especially for complex clients. This helps deepen the therapeutic relationship and allows the client to start forming new internal experiences of safety and connection.

This work can be deep and powerful; it helps clients start to heal the wounded inner child and co-construct meaning around their life experiences. It strengthens what Richard Schwartz in IFS would call the "Self," or what I refer to as the "Wise Self."

Once the client is resourced and more regulated—through attachment-based work and techniques like RDI—I begin trauma processing with EMDR.

## How has your approach to EMDR evolved since you first completed your training?

I felt an instant connection with EMDR from the moment I attended my basic training in 2009. It was clinically life-changing; I finally had a framework for case formulation through a trauma lens, which I could clearly explain to clients. Clients often said, "No one has ever explained it to me like that. It makes so much sense." The training I attended also hinted at spiritual integration, which felt like music to my soul. It gave me permission to begin weaving spirituality into my work more openly.

As I've previously mentioned, confidence in the standard protocol is essential. I continue to honor it fully, only adapting when clinically necessary and tailoring it to suit the developmental stage of each client.

A few years later, I trained in DDP, an attachment-based approach originally developed for adopted or fostered children. But its principles extend far beyond that; they can be applied in therapy with anyone and even inform interactions with friends, colleagues, and family. That training transformed my therapeutic relationships and gave me a stronger ability to formulate from both an attachment and trauma perspective—especially when integrating EMDR.

Learning parts work and ego state therapy early on was also essential—especially in supporting dissociative clients. It has since become a core component of my EMDR work, deepening as my knowledge and confidence have grown.

Another key area I've cultivated over time is narrative EMDR. Originally developed by Joan Lovett, this approach applies well to a broad range of clinical presentations in children, adolescents, and adults. It's a gentle and digestible way to introduce the core elements of EMDR, especially for adopted children, children in foster care, and refugees. It's also highly effective for complex adolescents and adults, or for those who are too dysregulated or hesitant to use the standard protocol. I've written trauma-informed, attachment-based, and transpersonal EMDR narratives to support clients during formulation and preparation.

When I started my independent practice in 2013, I finally felt free to honor my spirituality and integrate it safely and authentically into clinical work. I was formally trained in mindfulness, which has since become an integral part of my work. I've also presented on integrating mindfulness and EMDR at various conferences, webinars, and trainings.

I also developed Heart-Led Psychotherapy and began writing and teaching others how to integrate spirituality into EMDR. Adding a spiritual component to EMDR has enabled me to work with clients who seek to heal on a multidimensional, soul-based level, including work with past lives and soul retrieval. This remains one of the most profound aspects of both my EMDR journey and my overall career.

*Adding a spiritual component to EMDR has enabled me to work with clients who seek to heal on a multidimensional, soul-based level.*

## What self-care practices do you engage in regularly?

I'm passionate about integrating self-care into daily life. It's essential—not a luxury. That said, it's taken me many years to fully commit to my own healing and health.

Many therapists carry archetypes like the self-sacrificer, people-pleaser, martyr, or rescuer. They pour their energy into others, often at the expense of their own well-being. Of course, in life there are often real barriers to self-care, such as family demands, personal challenges, or unsupportive environments.

I found it easier to maintain self-care before I had children. Once they arrived, everything changed. I was constantly rushing—working, parenting two children (one with complex, undiagnosed neurodivergence), and managing a household—with barely any time for myself. I was so exhausted that, some nights, I didn't even have the energy to read them bedtime stories.

As a highly sensitive person with ADHD and dyslexic traits, my nervous system was either overstimulated or depleted. Even when I carved out time for yoga or a bike ride, I felt anxious about being away too long from my responsibilities. Looking back, I now see that I found spaciousness uncomfortable—even frightening—and filled it with endless doing. I wasn't committing to myself, perhaps out of fear of what that quiet space might reveal.

> *I found spaciousness uncomfortable—even frightening—and filled it with endless doing.*

Nearly 11 years later, I made significant changes. I left the NHS to work independently, then became a single parent, which brought its own stresses and financial pressures. But I also began living more mindfully and engaging in soul-level healing. It was powerful and transformative—and required me to devote more time to self-care to process and integrate the healing.

I still hear clinicians describe themselves as "busy," and it's often praised as a badge of honor. But sometimes "busy" is a way of avoiding self-care. That's not a judgment—just an observation, and one I've previously lived.

Self-care allows you to be authentic in your work, practicing what you preach. Have you ever paused to listen to the words you say to clients or to others? Try practicing this and reflect on how much of your advice you actually live yourself. Could those wise words be meant for you too? When we speak from our hearts and with authenticity, our words carry a higher energetic vibration and will have a greater impact on others.

> *When we speak from our hearts and with authenticity, our words carry a higher energetic vibration.*

During the COVID-19 pandemic, I prioritized two to three hours of self-care each day. That may sound like a lot—and it is—but I had to shift my belief system and take some big leaps of faith to align with my heart and soul. That time is the most important part of my day. It helps me operate at the energetic level I aspire to. It helps me regulate my nervous system and return to my window of tolerance—whether I feel activated or depleted.

I start each day with affirmations. Throughout the day, I utilize various tools to calm and regulate myself, including mindful breathing, meditation, heart coherence, nature walks, gardening, yoga, music, and mantras. Other practices—like pickleball, tennis, dance, and informal mindfulness—help clear stuck or heavy energy. I also regularly cleanse my energy and space using black sage, crystals, sound therapy, drumming, and Epsom salt baths.

I'm mindful of what I eat and drink, who I connect with, and the energy of my environment—and I adjust accordingly to support my physical, emotional, cognitive, and spiritual well-being. Finding moments of joy and play is essential, too.

## References

Dent, A. (2020). Using spirituality in psychotherapy: The heart led approach to clinical practice. Routledge.

Dent, A. (2021). Heart-led psychotherapy: A biopsychosocialspiritual model for clinical practice. Transpersonal Psychology Review, 23(1), 20–31.

Dent, A. (2025). Using spirituality in EMDR therapy: The heart led approach. Routledge.

Dobo, A.J. (2015). Unburdening souls at the speed of thought: Psychology, Christianity, and the transforming power of EMDR. Soul Psych Publishers.

Dobo, A.J. (2023). The hero's journey: Integrating Jungian psychology and EMDR therapy. Soul Psych Publishers.

Hacker Hughes, J. (2017). Towards a biopsychosociospiritual approach to psychological distress. Transpersonal Psychology Review, 19(1), 12–14.

Korn, D.L., and Leeds, A.M. (2002). Preliminary evidence of efficacy for EMDR resource development and installation in the stabilization phase of treatment of complex post traumatic disorder. Journal of Clinical Psychology, 58(12), 1465–1487.

Krystal, S., Prendergast, J., Krystal, P., Fenner, P., Shapiro, I., & Shapiro, K. (2002). Transpersonal psychology, Eastern nondual philosophy, and EMDR. In F. Shapiro (Ed.), EMDR as an integrative psychotherapy approach: Experts of diverse orientations explore the paradigm prism (pp. 319–339). American Psychological Association.

Logie, R.D.J., Bowers, M., Dent, A., Elliott, J., O'Connor, M., & Russell, A. (2020). Using Stories in EMDR: A guide to the storytelling (narrative) approach in EMDR therapy. From: Trauma Aid UK.

Lovett, J. (1999). Small wonders: Healing childhood trauma with EMDR. The Free Press.

Lovett, J. (2015). Trauma-attachment tangle. Modifying EMDR to help children resolve trauma and develop loving relationships. Routledge.

Parnell, L. (1996). Eye movement desensitization and reprocessing (EMDR) and spiritual unfolding. The Journal of Transpersonal Psychology, 28(2), 129–153. http://www.atpweb.org/jtparchive/trps-28-96-02-129.pdf

Rothschild, B. (2017). The Body Remembers (Volume 2): Revolutionizing Trauma Treatment. W.W. Norton & Company.

Shapiro, R. (2009). EMDR solutions II: For depression, eating disorders, performance and more. W.W. Norton & Company.

Siegel, I.R. (2017). The sacred path of the therapists: Modern healing, ancient wisdom, and client transformation. W.W. Norton & Company.

Siegel, I.R. (2018). EMDR as a transpersonal therapy: A trauma-focused approach to awakening consciousness. Journal of EMDR Practice and Research, 12(1), 24–43.

Van der Kolk, B. (2014). The body keeps the score: Brain, mind, and body in the healing of trauma. Penguin Books.

# Chapter 10

# Hypnosis Joins EMDR to Treat Chronic Pain: Mark Grant

As an Australian psychologist and researcher with 30 years of clinical experience, Mark Grant, MA, has become a key figure in developing trauma-informed treatments for chronic pain and persistent physical symptoms (PPS) using EMDR. He coauthored a chapter on EMDR treatment of pain for *The Oxford Handbook of EMDR Therapy*. Drawing on insights from dissociation, neurobiology, and somatic psychology, he developed a trauma-informed model that culminated in the evidence-based treatment manual *Pain Control with EMDR*. He has also created numerous self-help resources for people suffering from trauma and pain, including the Healing Traumatic Stress app series, which was the subject of the first randomized controlled trial of EMDR-based mobile apps.

Mark's identity has been shaped by diverse influences, including a Christian upbringing, an artist mother, an engineer father, struggles with ADHD, and a lifelong love of water from growing up on a small island at the bottom of the world, in New Zealand. He emigrated to Australia in 1981 and graduated as a psychologist in 1989.

Mark's interest in pain grew after discovering that there were a lack of effective psychological therapies for patients with chronic pain and PPS. Although Mark does not suffer from physical pain himself, being the eldest son of a chronic pain sufferer gave him a deep sensitivity to the needs of people living with chronic pain from an early age. He aspires to live a useful life. His wife, Ana, is also a clinical psychologist and a valuable partner in much of his work.

## Which books have influenced your work as a therapist?

***Uncommon Therapy: The Psychiatric Techniques of Milton H. Erickson, M.D.* by Jay Haley**

Before EMDR, Ericksonian hypnosis opened my eyes to the possibility of rapid, dramatic change in ways unimaginable with cognitive behavioral therapy, which dominated at the time. This witty and delightful collection of cases shows how a skilled clinician can transform seemingly intractable problems by delivering the right input at the right time. Erickson believed hypnotic trance creates a "break in a person's unconscious and habitual associations, so that creative learning can take place"—a definition that also fits EMDR.

However, trying to emulate Erickson proved daunting. Francine Shapiro's explanation of EMDR's processes offered a much clearer path to producing dramatic change without needing to become Erickson. That said, the standard EMDR trauma protocol soon required significant modifications to address issues such as chronic pain and dissociative disorders.

***EMDR as an Integrative Psychotherapy: Experts of Diverse Orientations Explore the Paradigm Prism* edited by Francine Shapiro**

This collection of articles on how EMDR integrates with other approaches is one of my most frequently referenced texts. This book reminds me that EMDR is more than the eight phases. It offers a range of methods that contribute to EMDR and can be called upon when standard EMDR proves ineffective. This text paved the way for me to integrate hypnosis into EMDR treatment of chronic pain and somatic symptoms. Trauma processing alone is often insufficient for these patients, many of whom also suffer from medical illnesses or serious injuries. Hypnosis helps build resources to manage persistent somatic symptoms.

***Memories, Dreams, Reflections* by Carl G. Jung**

Jung's seminal work highlights core therapeutic themes: life as a journey toward individuation, the power of dreams, and the importance of embracing the unconscious. He stresses following one's inner voice, even when it strays from conventional paths, and the transformative potential of confronting the shadow self. These themes anticipated the current recognition of dissociation and ego state approaches. Jung's memoir reminds me that therapy is about much more than trauma processing.

Avi, a young man with strong Christian faith, was traumatized by the sacrifices he had made to rescue his family from financial ruin. His inability to complete tertiary studies left him feeling inferior in his chosen occupation as a health coach. Under the stress of the family situation, Avi had used drugs several years earlier, which triggered a drug-induced psychosis and a traumatic stay as an inpatient at a psychiatric facility—an event that scarred him.

After many months of therapy, including EMDR, Avi described a recent conflict with his sister over his role in rescuing the family. I had a hunch there was an unacknowledged part carrying deep sadness about the toll this had taken. I asked, "If you could speak to that self now, what would you say?" Avi immediately teared up and chokingly replied, "That experience was meant for me—it took everything, but I did it." He added, "God, my family, and friends were with me." Avi could now separate himself from the effects of what had happened, see how he had grown through it, embrace his faith, and recognize it as part of life's journey.

## How do you explain EMDR to your clients?

Most patients now arrive with at least a basic awareness of EMDR, unlike when I started in the early 1990s. My explanation depends on each patient's needs; some seek a detailed understanding, others want to proceed with therapy. My explanations unfold gradually, often referencing the adaptive information processing (AIP) model or neuroplasticity, as appropriate. I say something along the lines of:

*EMDR works by "hijacking" the fight-or-flight response—diverting attention from traumatic memories to bilateral stimulation (BLS). This shift triggers a relaxation response, which becomes linked to the memory. Everyone has an orienting response: Our attention is naturally drawn to novel external stimuli. So, when recalling trauma (internal stimuli) and noticing BLS (external stimuli), your attention shifts involuntarily. This survival mechanism keeps you safe; in EMDR, we deliberately activate it instead of being overwhelmed by trauma.*

This explanation integrates brain functioning, the AIP model, and Erickson's concept of utilization—EMDR is harnessing an innate survival response.

## What advice do you have for new EMDR therapists?

**Understand that learning and skill unfold over time.** Having learned one of the most powerful tools in psychology, you are now faced with the challenge of integrating EMDR with your existing knowledge and figuring out how to use that tool safely and effectively. As you continue to practice, you will get a sense of when, where, and how to use EMDR, as well as its limitations. You will learn that no therapy works for everyone, every time.

**Get to know your patients.** For anything but the simplest PTSD, you must know your patient reasonably well, which comes only from spending time with them and gathering information—not only their trauma history but also their attachment history and personality traits. As the old adage goes, "It's more important to know what patient has the disease than what disease the patient has."

*As the old adage goes, "It's more important to know what patient has the disease than what disease the patient has."*

**Be ready when the patient is ready.** Have the courage to begin processing as soon as the patient is ready, not necessarily after you have ticked all the boxes of a perfect case conceptualization. After many months of treating a chronic pain sufferer, I was told by a client that whenever her husband was away on business, she went to sleep clutching a scrap of silk salvaged from a childhood wrap. This "scrap" of information told me more about her anxieties and the impact of loss of control from pain than all the trauma questionnaires ever could. After that I focused on her inner security more than pain.

**Get comfortable with abreactions.** We therapists are, in many ways, wounded healers. You need to be comfortable with abreactions and spontaneous emotional expression. This will be much easier if you have done some of your own work.

**Learn from your mistakes.** You will make mistakes—that's part of learning anything new. If you are an ethical, competent therapist, your mistakes will contribute to your learning and do no great harm.

## What is one therapeutic approach that integrates really well with EMDR?

It's a hard choice between somatic psychology and hypnosis for my favorite complementary approach, but I'd pick hypnosis. Hypnosis is not so much a method as it is a tool for delivering therapy, like a syringe used to deliver medication. Recalling Erickson's definition of hypnosis—a "break in a person's unconscious and habitual associations, so that creative learning can take place"—EMDR relies on numerous hypnotic processes, for example, induction, age regression/progression, and trance ratification. This makes hypnosis a natural adjunct to EMDR.

> *Hypnosis is a tool for delivering therapy,*
> *like a syringe used to deliver medication.*

The entire EMDR setup, including dual attention and bilateral stimulation, can be viewed as a form of induction aimed at inducing an altered state of consciousness, where the patient becomes more receptive to new possibilities or ways of thinking. The difference is that EMDR relies on linking the positive changes to the PC rather than giving suggestions.

Another similarity is the EMDR floatback (age regression) and the future template (age progression). The EMDR check-in is essentially a form of trance ratification, where the patient's attention is drawn to phenomenological changes that affirm that change is happening. It's no coincidence that Francine Shapiro was trained in neurolinguistic programming before developing EMDR.

Here are three ways in which hypnosis can complement EMDR:

**Hypnosis enhances your ability to utilize EMDR processes.** For example, it helps if you make changes explicit during the EMDR check-in, without overdoing it. The ability to notice physiological changes following BLS, which can be quite subtle when treating chronic pain or PPS, is the foundation on which change evolves.

Many patients enter a trance state in which they experience relaxation and free association, following desensitization, during which they are very receptive to suggestion. Limiting this state to simply installing a positive cognition (PC) may be a wasted opportunity for a patient who needs to develop a deeper, broader sense of their self-worth.

Adding suggestions to the installation process (for example, "You can enjoy the feeling of well-being that comes from realizing you are lovable, strong, worthwhile—feeling that in your body now...) can greatly enhance the adoption of more positive self-states.

**Hypnosis enhances your ability to utilize the therapeutic relationship.** As Erickson once said, "Although the individual is the unit of change, it is the therapeutic relationship that ignites the transformation process." As EMDR has evolved to address more complex presentations, the importance of the therapeutic relationship is increasingly recognized. The attunement that lies at the heart of the therapeutic relationship is key to almost every aspect of EMDR, from target selection to pacing to repairing attachment wounds. Attunement facilitates safety, openness, and relational capacities, both internal and external.

**Imagery can be delivered hypnotically.** This is essential as a resourcing strategy for symptom management, particularly when treating persistent pain. This involves the delivery of more curated imaginal resources (for example, antidote imagery, healing resources, or employing dissociative strategies). See my book *Pain Control with EMDR* for more details.

I believe that training in hypnosis, even if only a workshop or two, will enhance your skills as a therapist, regardless of the modalities you are employing. The American Society of Clinical Hypnosis offers numerous training programs and self-guided learning opportunities.

> *Training in hypnosis, even if only a workshop or two, will enhance your skills as a therapist.*

## What role does attachment theory play in your EMDR practice?

Attachment is essential for healthy mind-body development, shaping brain systems for self-regulation and stress management. We know that attachment problems predispose people to PTSD, pain, and disease. The attachment-diathesis model of chronic pain links insecure attachment to greater vulnerability to chronic pain via stress dysregulation, altered immune responses, and maladaptive coping patterns. This model also informs treatment.

An understanding of attachment processes and how they can be disrupted by trauma is vital to understanding the impact of trauma and negotiating the relationship between trauma and pain or PPS therapeutically. Here is a brief introduction to attachment and its relevance to therapy.

*An understanding of attachment processes and how they can be disrupted by trauma is vital.*

## The Neuroscience of Attachment Theory

Attachment is mediated by several key brain systems:

- **The reward system (mesolimbic system):** This system involves the prefrontal cortex, amygdala, and hippocampus, driven by neurotransmitters such as dopamine, GABA, and oxytocin. Secure attachment activates this system, promoting pleasure, bonding, and stress regulation. Mothers with abuse histories often have lower oxytocin, affecting both mother and child.

- **Novelty pathway (ventral striatal):** This pathway is dominant early in life, driving exploration.

- **Familiarity pathway (dorsal striatal):** This pathway develops through secure caregiving, fostering comfort and safety. Abuse or neglect inhibits the development of the dorsal pathway, leaving the novelty-seeking pathway dominant, which can predispose individuals to risk-taking and substance abuse.

- **The HPA axis (hypothalamic-pituitary-adrenal):** This system regulates stress via cortisol. Early trauma hyperactivates the HPA axis, increasing cortisol and impairing hippocampal development, which further reduces stress-regulation capacity. The amygdala becomes hypersensitive, leading to increased fear and vigilance.

Neglect or abuse shifts brain development toward heightened novelty-seeking and impaired comfort-safety preferences. Infants may still bond with abusive caregivers due to early neurobiological imprinting. Stress elevates amygdala activity and cortisol, disrupting self-regulation. Insecure attachment is linked to lower brain-derived neurotrophic factor in the prefrontal cortex, reducing the brain's ability to regulate fear responses.

## Cortisol, Health, and Pain

The HPA axis interacts with the immune system in the following ways:

- Acute cortisol increases help reduce inflammation.
- Chronic cortisol elevation, however, increases inflammation and raises risks for autoimmune diseases, cardiovascular problems, gastrointestinal disorders, pain syndromes, and cancer.
- Insecurely attached adults have heightened cortisol reactivity and are less likely to seek social support under stress. Pain itself activates the HPA axis; chronic severe pain can cause cortisol dysregulation, worsening pain and impairing healing. Hormonal changes (for example, DHEA, progesterone, or thyroid) further influence pain regulation. Persistent hypercortisolism contributes to bone and joint degeneration, while low cortisol (hypocortisolism) leads to weakness and low blood pressure.

## Therapeutic Relationship in Healing

Understanding the role of attachment problems in stress reminds us that, in all but the most straightforward cases, the therapeutic relationship is central. Core competencies include:

- Clear therapeutic intent
- Attunement and analytic listening
- Working within relational dynamics
- Pattern recognition and linking
- Navigating ruptures and repairs
- Courageous, disciplined communication

In EMDR, the therapist facilitates reactivation of the AIP system without imposing content and while ensuring emotional safety. The latter is facilitated through attunement, evaluation of client readiness, and resourcing as necessary. Shapiro emphasized that accessible positive memory networks, including those formed in therapy, are prerequisites for effective reprocessing.

> *Accessible positive memory networks, including those formed in therapy, are prerequisites for effective reprocessing.*

EMDR is a sensitive psychotherapy, requiring:

- **Timing:** using attunement as part of assessing readiness for processing
- **Being client-centered:** adjusting BLS type and speed
- **Pacing:** balancing facilitation with allowing client-led processing
- **Awareness:** noticing transference and countertransference, especially with disorganized attachment

You can watch my YouTube explainer video, "A 3-Step Trauma-Informed Approach to Overcoming Pain," which summarizes the relationship between attachment problems, trauma, and pain.

## What creative modifications have you made to EMDR to address specific populations or presenting issues?

While trauma and chronic pain or PPS share many overlaps, key differences—such as organic pathology, nociplastic pain, and medical trauma—require tailored adaptations to the standard EMDR trauma protocol. Adjustments remain consistent with EMDR principles when supported by sound rationale or research.

Here are 10 pain protocol variations to the standard EMDR trauma protocol for chronic pain or persistent physical symptoms that I have developed and researched during the past 30 years. I also want to acknowledge Bruce Eimer as an inspiration and originator of several of these variations.

- **Pain history:** As in PTSD work, EMDR history taking for chronic pain or PPS should screen for trauma but also recognize that not all pain is trauma related. In addition, physical pathology associated with injury or disease processes may also be a contributing factor. Many clients present with mixed histories of trauma, neglect, health problems, and extensive medical interventions, which themselves may cause trauma (for instance, surgery recipients have higher PTSD rates). A thorough medical history—including childhood illness, hospitalizations, and current health beliefs—is essential.

- **Health status:** The AIP model assumes innate healing capacity, but chronic illness or injury can limit readiness for EMDR's demands. Assessing overall health and energy is a vital part of phase 2, ensuring clients can engage with traumatic material without becoming energetically overwhelmed.

- **Resourcing:** Resourcing takes on a stronger somatic focus for pain or PPS clients. Strategies include imagery for pain relief, accessing memories of comfort, and distraction. Relief felt after BLS can be transformed into "antidote imagery" and installed with BLS or hypnosis. Exhausted clients may need energy-enhancing and affect-regulation resources, such as relaxation techniques, safe-place imagery, and positive memory networks. Pain-focused resources, future templates, and hypnotic inductions aimed at healing and coping are necessary in most cases.

- **EMDR targeting:** Targets may include past trauma, present pain, or the effects of pain. Present pain is often the priority, as it can feel like an internal threat that compromises safety. Targeting present pain aids in stabilization and mastery. Where there is no direct trauma, imagery may be based on sensory descriptors, such as size, shape, or color of pain. If both trauma and pain are present, the client chooses which to address first.

- **Substituting sensations for emotions:** When focusing on present pain, physical sensations can replace emotional states in the EMDR target setup. The sensation itself serves as the negative affect. This avoids unnecessary complexity and keeps the focus on reprocessing the pain experience.

> *The sensation itself serves as the negative affect.*

- **Negative and positive cognitions:** Trauma survivors often endorse NCs about safety and control, whereas pain clients lean toward themes of responsibility and defectiveness. Chronic pain sufferers may struggle to believe PCs early on; it is often better to introduce PCs after some pain relief is achieved, making them easier to accept (for example, "I can cope" or "I can control the pain").

- **Continuous audio BLS:** Unlike standard practice, continuous BLS without frequent pauses can be helpful in pain work, allowing gradual, subtle changes to accumulate. Check-ins occur every 30 to 60 seconds or when nonverbal shifts are noted. Auditory BLS is especially useful, possibly tapping into deeper subcortical processing, and can be used between sessions for self-soothing.

- **Tracking and facilitating BLS effects:** Clients may not notice subtle changes due to dissociation or alexithymia. Therapists should monitor both verbal and nonverbal cues, and direct awareness to bodily changes. Positive shifts can be reinforced with BLS or hypnotic suggestions to integrate new, more comfortable states into daily life.

- **Self-use of BLS:** For appropriate clients, audio BLS at home can be a safe, effective tool for reducing pain, stress, and insomnia. It should be introduced only after in-session positive experiences with BLS and framed as self-soothing rather than self-administered EMDR. I created four apps addressing four key symptoms of PTSD: pain, insomnia, anxiety, and sleep, which can be found in my Healing Traumatic Stress app series. A pilot study of these apps suggests that self-use of BLS, coupled with guided hypnotic suggestions, could significantly reduce PTSD symptoms and associated health issues.

- **Hypnosis:** In addition to facilitating standard EMDR, hypnosis enables the installation of healing resources for managing persistent pain. Some of my favorite inductions include "antidote imagery," unconscious activation of healing resources, ideomotor signaling for processing unconscious conflicts, utilizing dissociation, and memory work. See my treatment manual or my website (h ttps://www.overcomingpain.com) for more hypnotic scripts.

**Case example:** A highly intelligent young medical professional sought help coping with chronic pain stemming from a leg injury. Due to the emotional effects of being raised in a harsh emotional environment with high family expectations, Jeff had initially ignored the injury and continued working very hard in an attempt to regain control of his life. Jeff's coping strategy consisted of setting incremental but ever-higher goals for himself in the hope that he could work through the pain.

By the time he sought treatment from me, he could barely walk and was confined to his bed for 23 hours a day. Jeff was depressed as a result of having to postpone marrying his girlfriend and having a family, as well as the negative effects on his career goals. The combination of attachment trauma, disabling uncontrolled pain, trauma associated with the effects of his pain, ineffective medical treatments, and his personality demanded a flexible, integrated approach incorporating most of the above variations.

Following three years of treatment incorporating the EMDR protocol and adjunctive approaches, such as hypnosis and ego-state work targeting a harsh inner critic, Jeff was not completely pain-free, but he could walk five kilometers, he could work in a normal environment, and he was able to get married and start a family.

**Conclusion:** After PTSD, pain is the most researched application of EMDR. While EMDR principles remain intact, chronic pain and PPS cases benefit from specific, research-informed modifications in history taking, readiness assessment, resource development, target selection, and use of BLS—particularly in addressing the unique somatic and cognitive aspects of pain.

I've also found that many people ultimately grow psychologically and spiritually through suffering, and I hold space for these larger, transcendent possibilities when patients are open to them. We are much more than our problems. As others have alluded to in this book, there is a tension in EMDR between method and psychodynamic and spiritual elements of healing. It's worth remembering that the original meaning of the word "healing" is to make whole.

## What self-care practices do you engage in regularly?

I used to enjoy an alcoholic beverage at the end of my working day to relax and dull my mind from the stimulation of my work. However, my evening drink became a habitual numbing strategy that masked my insufficient attention to the need for rest and regeneration.

After a combination of personal reflection and a random conversation with a life coach at a conference, I replaced my evening drink with yoga and incorporated more self-care time into my life. I feel so much more balanced and even proud of breaking such a long-standing habit.

The basics of self-care—pacing your workload, exercise, recreation, and more— are generally understood; although, as with any behavior, it all starts with attitude. Do you feel like your needs matter? How do you balance your needs against the needs of your patients? What do you do to maintain self-awareness around your needs?

> *Do you feel like your needs matter? What do you do to maintain self-awareness around your needs?*

Working with EMDR poses unique challenges for self-care, particularly in the following scenarios:

You will be working with more trauma, which is inherently more emotionally demanding than treating something like a simple phobia. You will encounter dissociation, relational complexities, and blockages.

Patients often enter EMDR therapy with expectations of rapid treatment results, which may not be possible with more complex presentations—as most cases involving pain or somatization are. It's essential to maintain your boundaries, recognize your limitations, and avoid taking on too much responsibility.

Seek out therapy for yourself. Knowing yourself and addressing your own trauma will protect you from burnout.

## References

Grant, M. (2009). Pain control with EMDR. Overcoming Pain. https://www.overcomingpain.com/pain-control-with-emdr

Grant, M., Lau, R. C., & DiNardo, J. (2025). Feasibility and potential efficacy of a mobile app series based on eye movement desensitization and reprocessing: A pilot randomized controlled trial with posttraumatic stress disorder and comorbid problems. Journal of EMDR Practice and Research, 19, Article 0003.

Grant, M., & Tesarz, J. (2025). EMDR in somatization and persistent physical symptoms. In D. Farrell, S. J. Schubert, & M. D. Kiernan (Eds.), The Oxford handbook of EMDR therapy. Oxford University Press.

Haley, J. (1973). Uncommon therapy: The psychiatric techniques of Milton H. Erickson, M.D. W.W. Norton & Company.

Jung, C. G. (1989). Memories, dreams, reflections (A. Jaffé, Ed.; R. Winston & C. Winston, Trans.; Rev. ed.). Vintage Books.

Shapiro, F. (Ed.). (2002). EMDR as an integrative psychotherapy: Experts of diverse orientations explore the paradigm prism. American Psychological Association.

# Chapter 11

# EMDR and Parts Work: Luna Medina-Wolf

Luna Medina-Wolf, MEd, LMHC, NCC, MCAP, is an EMDRIA-approved consultant, EMDR part 1 trainer with EMDR HAP, and a qualified supervisor in Florida. She is the owner of Helping Moon Counseling, a group practice in Boca Raton specializing in trauma and healing. Luna was the 2025–2026 president of the Mental Health Counselor Association of Palm Beach.

Fluent in English, Spanish, and Hebrew, Luna brings a culturally attuned and inclusive approach to her work. She has extensive experience supporting individuals navigating trauma, anxiety, and substance use, and is recognized for her warmth, presence, and commitment to her clients' healing.

Her enthusiasm for EMDR therapy ignited on the second day of her basic training and has deepened through years of advanced study and consultation. She is particularly interested in blending dissociation work within EMDR's phased methodology and is convinced of its ability to drive lasting transformation.

Luna is a past recipient of the Florida Counseling Association Member of the Year Award and the Florida Mental Health Counselors Association Advocate of the Year Award.

## Which books have influenced your work as a therapist?

***Easy Ego State Interventions: Strategies for Working with Parts* by Robin Shapiro**

This is one of the most influential books in my development as a therapist. I've always been drawn to inner child work, but didn't receive formal training in it early on. After discovering EMDR in 2016, I focused on strengthening my skills as a trauma clinician. This book opened the door to integrating parts work into my EMDR practice in a way that felt both practical and accessible. It motivated me to pursue additional training in ego state and parts-based models.

The case examples and user-friendly scripts helped me implement techniques right away, and this integration has brought greater fluidity and effectiveness to my EMDR sessions, especially with complex and dissociative clients.

***The Polyvagal Theory in Therapy: Engaging the Rhythm of Regulation* by Deb Dana**

This book is another foundational text in my growth as a therapist. I believe that every client should leave therapy with concrete tools to regulate their nervous system and build resilience. Early in my career, I spent significant time learning grounding and resourcing techniques, but Deb Dana's work, along with Stephen Porges's research, gave me a clear, science-based framework that tied it all together.

Understanding the autonomic nervous system and the role of safety in the therapeutic relationship has been transformational. Her worksheets and interventions help my clients cultivate self-awareness and regulation, and they've become a core part of my resourcing and preparation phases in EMDR.

***The Body Keeps the Score: Brain, Mind, and Body in the Healing of Trauma* by Bessel van der Kolk**

Like many therapists, my own life experiences brought me to this work. I've done the personal healing required to be present for others, but this book reminded me that growth is ongoing—and that healing is possible not just for clients, but for ourselves too. It validated the importance of trauma-informed care and reinforced my belief in the mind-body connection. Though more clinical in tone, I often recommend it to clients who want a deeper understanding of their trauma.

Each of these books broadened my outlook, strengthened my skills, and fueled my passion for trauma healing, particularly through the lens of EMDR therapy.

## How do you explain EMDR to your clients?

I describe EMDR by saying something along the lines of:

*EMDR is a comprehensive therapy that helps people heal from difficult or traumatic experiences by changing how those memories affect them today. EMDR works by identifying distressing memories and guiding the brain to process them in a different way, so they have a reduced emotional impact.*

*When we bring these memories up in a supportive environment, EMDR enables the brain to naturally process them. Instead of replaying a memory exactly the same way each time, the brain has a chance to update it, much like adjusting the story a little with every retelling.*

*EMDR utilizes this natural brain mechanism to update memories with more accurate and adaptive information. Over time, this reduces the emotional intensity of the memory and shifts the beliefs, emotions, and body responses associated with it—what we call a "state change."*

*If you cut your arm and it's clean, your body knows how to heal it. But if there's dirt, bacteria, or the wound is too deep, it needs help—maybe stitches or antiseptics. EMDR is like that kind of help, but for the brain.*

*After a traumatic experience, the brain may struggle to fully process what happened. This leaves the person stuck with distressing feelings and beliefs. EMDR enables the brain to access the information it needs to resolve those experiences and resume its natural healing process.*

*In sessions, we focus on the components of memory—images, thoughts, emotions, and body sensations—and how they're connected. EMDR utilizes structured protocols and bilateral stimulation, such as eye movements, to help link distressing memories to more adaptive information, allowing these memories to no longer feel stuck, triggering, or overwhelming.*

*Ultimately, EMDR helps you shift your perception of the memory, creating lasting relief and emotional freedom.*

## What is one therapeutic approach that integrates really well with EMDR?

In my view, one of the most powerful therapeutic approaches that integrates seamlessly with EMDR is ego state therapy. When working with trauma, dissociation isn't just common; it's expected. Yet it's often overlooked in graduate programs and, until recently, received little emphasis in clinical training, including basic EMDR training.

After nearly 10 years of practicing EMDR, I am convinced that understanding dissociation and parts work is vital to being an effective EMDR therapist. Ego state therapy, Internal Family Systems (IFS), and related models offer a structured, compassionate framework for engaging with internal parts that frequently arise during trauma treatment.

> *Understanding dissociation and parts work is vital to being an effective EMDR therapist.*

Without this foundation, clinicians may face repeated blocks, looping, or even re-traumatization, especially with complex trauma and early attachment wounds. Some of my most impactful learning experiences have come from experts such as Robin Shapiro, Dolores Mosquera, Kathy Steele, Jim Knipe, Shirley Jean Schmidt, and others. Their work has helped me bring greater depth, nuance, and safety into my sessions.

Before learning ego state therapy, I often felt stuck with complex cases, especially those involving early trauma. Even after solid phase 2 preparation, I sometimes hit a wall—blocked processing or clients feeling "stuck." After adding ego state work, I could better identify and work with protective or wounded parts, making processing smoother and safer.

One case stands out clearly. A 35-year-old woman was referred for EMDR to address a memory of sexual molestation from age eight. Doriana had also developed a stutter around the same time. We completed phases 1 and 2, and she responded well to resourcing, utilizing tools such as the container, safe place, and healing imagery. We also identified and established communication with several parts, including a dominant protector. All parts gave consent to begin reprocessing, and Doriana consistently practiced her tools between sessions.

Initially, reprocessing proceeded smoothly, and she maintained good dual awareness. But toward the end of one session, something shifted. Doriana became emotionally detached, saying things like, "Nothing is coming up" and "I feel kind of numb." It was clear she was dissociating.

Thanks to my ego state training, I knew how to respond. I gently invited her to check in with the part that felt numb. Somewhat surprised, Doriana paused and said, "I don't think we should continue. It's too much."

We changed focus and spent several sessions strengthening the rapport between her adult self and the younger, traumatized part. As trust grew, the younger part revealed that the abuse was ongoing, not just a single incident. Though understandably overwhelming at first, this insight allowed her to fully engage in EMDR reprocessing. Doriana was able to desensitize the memory—and notably, her stutter significantly improved.

This case illustrates how ego state therapy promotes safety, structure, and insight, facilitating deeper EMDR work. For clinicians who treat complex trauma, integrating parts work is not just beneficial; it is essential.

> *Ego state therapy promotes safety, structure, and insight, facilitating deeper EMDR work.*

## What EMDR success story caught you by surprise?

The success story I want to share comes from my work through the Trauma Recovery Network (TRN) chapter of EMDR HAP. On February 14, 2018, everything changed for so many in our South Florida community, particularly in Coral Springs and Parkland. A tragic school shooting at Marjory Stoneman Douglas High School took the lives of 17 people and injured 17 others.

It was a devastating loss—one that deeply shook our entire region. I had been practicing EMDR for a few years at that point, but I had never encountered anything like this.

Our local TRN chapter hosted a training on an early EMDR intervention called the Recent Traumatic Episode Protocol (RTEP/GTEP). That training changed my life—and the lives of so many people I had the privilege of working with.

> *The Recent Traumatic Episode Protocol (RTEP/GTEP) changed my life—and the lives of so many people I had the privilege of working with.*

When I began using this protocol, I wasn't sure what to expect. We were asked to offer three to five 90-minute pro bono sessions to those affected. We used the PCL-5 PTSD symptom scale to assess clients before and after treatment, evaluating their progress. I remember thinking, "Only five sessions to treat trauma from something this big?" But I chose to trust the model. I jumped in—consultant on speed dial—and started offering it.

I worked with many students, staff, and families from the school—and I was amazed by how effective the protocol was for so many of them. For those without prior trauma histories, I saw significant improvement, even after the first session. Many only needed two or three sessions. Most didn't even require all five.

For others with more complex histories, progress was slower—but still far faster and more effective than I ever expected in the aftermath of such a tragedy. I was so surprised by the results that I called several clients monthly for six months after our last session, just to make sure the progress had held. Many were still symptom-free.

That's when I truly understood the power EMDR holds. It became the heart of my work. I fully immersed myself in the model because I saw firsthand that it was the most effective way to help my clients. I also learned the importance of having a strong professional community. That support was essential while doing this kind of work.

My mentor, Deb Del Vecchio-Scully, was a guiding light throughout our journey. I started a peer support group for local therapists that continues to be a meaningful part of my life today.

It was a healing experience for them—and for me. I feel deeply honored to have been part of their journey. I strongly encourage all therapists to pursue training in early EMDR interventions. You never know when your community might be affected by a crisis—and when your skills might be exactly what's needed.

*You never know when your community might be affected by a crisis—and when your skills might be exactly what's needed.*

## How has your approach to EMDR evolved since you first completed your training?

When I first trained in EMDR nearly a decade ago, the landscape looked very different. Since then, the field has evolved in powerful and exciting ways, including the addition of a fourth theme, Connection and Belonging, introduced in 2021.

There's now a stronger emphasis on dissociation in basic training. And we've come to view the first two phases of EMDR not as rigid steps, but more like strands of a braid, as things we can fluidly weave between to meet each client's unique needs.

*We've come to view the first two phases of EMDR not as rigid steps, but more like strands of a braid, as things we can fluidly weave between to meet each client's unique needs.*

After my initial EMDR training, I explored a variety of trauma-focused modalities; I was curious and eager to offer my clients the best care possible. But no matter what I tried, I kept returning to EMDR. Its adaptability and depth continued to call me back.

While early critiques framed EMDR as rigid or overly "scripted," I learned that this perception missed the heart of the model. As one of my mentors, April Minjarez, beautifully says, "EMDR is client-centered, therapist-led." That framework allows us to meet clients with empathy and presence, while still gently guiding them toward adaptive resolution.

As I worked with more complex trauma cases, I realized how critical it was to deepen my understanding of dissociation. That insight changed everything. I immersed myself in learning from leaders like Robin Shapiro, Dolores Mosquera, and others. That journey led me to integrate ego state therapy into most of my work, and it's become one of the most valuable additions to my practice. Parts work has transformed my ability to guide clients through the EMDR phases, especially those with early or complex trauma histories.

Although my clinical tool kit has expanded, the core of my work remains rooted in the effectiveness of the standard EMDR protocol.

Over the years, many new protocols and adaptations have been developed—many of them excellent. Like others, I explored several, looking for the next best thing. But I've come to trust that the standard protocol, when applied thoughtfully and with attunement, contains everything we need. I occasionally draw from other protocols when appropriate, but more often than not, I rely on the foundational approach for its flexibility, structure, and effectiveness.

Ultimately, my EMDR practice has evolved through continued learning, mentorship, and experience. But the heart of it—trusting the process, honoring the client's pace, and using the standard protocol as a solid guide—has remained constant.

## Have you experienced imposter syndrome?

Absolutely. I experienced imposter syndrome when I first started practicing EMDR. To be honest, I still do from time to time. I often remind my consultees that questioning their abilities can actually be a sign of genuine care and a desire to grow. That mindset—the willingness to reflect and improve—is what enables us to become stronger and more effective therapists.

Initially, EMDR felt overwhelming. There were numerous components to track, and each client presented a unique set of challenges. I often found myself second-guessing whether I was doing it right or if I could have done it better.

What helped me most was practice and, more important, consultation. I'm incredibly grateful for every consultant who supported me along the way, especially as I worked toward becoming an EMDR trainer. Regular consultation gave me grounding and direction. It didn't erase imposter syndrome, but it gave me the tools, perspective, and reassurance I needed. Having someone to guide, encourage, and teach in real time is invaluable.

I've come to believe that imposter syndrome can be a motivator. It pushes us to stay curious, ask questions, and stay open to learning. With EMDR, there's always more to learn—and that's part of what makes it so powerful. Staying connected to a community, continuing education, and staying current with research are all ways I've built confidence and stayed inspired in this work.

You don't have to be perfect to be effective. You simply need to remain committed to learning, growing, and consistently showing up for your clients with humility, empathy, and skill.

*You don't have to be perfect to be effective.*

## What self-care practices do you engage in regularly?

As therapists, we give a great deal of ourselves to support others. Having an intentional self-care plan isn't just helpful; it's essential. The phrase "You can't pour from an empty cup" resonates deeply, especially for trauma therapists. We're often exposed to emotionally intense, sometimes disturbing material, which can gradually wear on both body and spirit. Without consistent self-care, burnout becomes a real risk.

One of my foundational practices is gratitude. Each morning, I begin the day with a moment of connection to myself and my higher self. I express thanks for my health, my family, the privilege of doing meaningful work, and anything else that comes to heart. I ask for strength to continue serving others. I close each day the same way, grounded in gratitude.

I also rely on aromatherapy. I start each morning with a calming essential oil blend in my diffuser and apply it topically throughout the day as needed, especially after emotionally heavy sessions.

Movement and laughter are powerful regulators for me. I often have impromptu dance parties with my kids after work to shake off the day and reconnect with joy.

Regular connection with my peer group is another vital support. Discussing clinical cases and sharing experiences with like-minded professionals nourishes me and reminds me I'm not alone in this work.

I also make space for physical care, including monthly massages with essential oils, regular manicures and pedicures, and any other treatments that help my body release tension. A shower or swim often helps when I feel heavy mentally or physically.

And when I notice signs of emotional overwhelm, I reach out to my own EMDR therapist for a tune-up session. That personal support is incredibly grounding.

These practices allow me to stay present, centered, and compassionate—not just for my clients, but for myself and my loved ones.

## References

Dana, D. (2018). The polyvagal theory in therapy: Engaging the rhythm of regulation. W. W. Norton & Company.

Porges, S. W. (2011). The polyvagal theory: Neurophysiological foundations of emotions, attachment, communication, and self-regulation. W. W. Norton & Company.

Shapiro, E., & Laub, B. (2008). Early EMDR intervention (EEI): A summary, a theoretical model, and the recent traumatic episode protocol (R-TEP). Journal of EMDR Practice and Research, 2(2), 79–96.

Shapiro, F. (2018). Eye movement desensitization and reprocessing (EMDR) therapy: Basic principles, protocols, and procedures (3rd ed.). Guilford Press.

Shapiro, R. (2016). Easy ego state interventions: Strategies for working with parts. W. W. Norton & Company.

van der Kolk, B. A. (2014). The body keeps the score: Brain, mind, and body in the healing of trauma. Penguin Books.

Weathers, F. W., Litz, B. T., Keane, T. M., Palmieri, P. A., Marx, B. P., & Schnurr, P. P. (2013). The PTSD Checklist for DSM-5 (PCL-5). National Center for PTSD.

# Chapter 12

# EMDR and IFS: David Polidi

David Polidi, MSW, MEd, LICSW, is an EMDRIA consultant-in-training, and a level 2–trained Internal Family Systems (IFS) therapist through the IFS Institute. He holds advanced training in Intimacy from the Inside Out and serves as a guide for The Syzygy Institute trainings.

Since 2000, David has worked with children and families in schools and community settings. Alongside his wife, who is also a licensed social worker, he cofounded Empowered Through Compassion, a practice offering trauma-informed therapy, couples counseling, and EMDR consultation across Massachusetts and New Hampshire.

David also hosts the podcast *Empowered Through Compassion*, where he interviews thought leaders in the healing professions and explores the natural synergy between EMDR and IFS, as well as other integrative approaches to inner work.

## Which books have influenced your work as a therapist?

***Listening Deeply* by Stephen R. Andrew**

In this concise and practical book, Andrew—a storyteller, trainer, coach, and consultant—begins by stating a central belief: True change is fostered through the heart, not the mind. The book offers valuable insights and consistently reflects his empathy. He encourages readers to approach therapy models with openness, emphasizing collaboration by joining clients in their pain with compassion, not with an urge to fix.

***The Art and Science of EMDR: Helping Clinicians Bridge the Path from Protocol to Practice* by Rotem Brayer**

This book explores how EMDR combines art and science, echoing Andrew's themes about balancing the heart and mind. Andrew suggests leading with empathy, and Brayer's work demonstrates that EMDR can become an expressive and creative process. Intuition and creativity help build deep trust with clients.

***Cradled in the Arms of Compassion: A Spiritual Journey from Trauma to Recovery* by Frank Rogers Jr.**

This book shares the story of one man's spiritual journey to healing. Rogers's message is about hope, love, and the healing he wished he could have offered his sister. Despite his efforts to care for his sister during her struggle with severe depression, she ultimately took her own life.

***IFS-Informed EMDR: Creative and Collaborative Approaches* edited by David Polidi**

Not being able to limit influential books to just three, I include this fourth volume, which features contributions from 22 leaders in trauma healing who have successfully integrated IFS and EMDR in clinical work and training. In this book, the reader is introduced to the foundations of EMDR and IFS as separate, transformative healing models.

Then, readers explore specific approaches that integrate EMDR with IFS and parts work, including Annabel McGoldrick's IFS-informed EMDR; the Syzygy model, described by its creator, Bruce Hersey; and the trauma-informed stabilization treatment model, shared by its founder, Janina Fisher. A later section presents frameworks such as somatic integration and processing, antiracist psychotherapy, structural dissociation, art therapy from a Jungian view, and spiritual perspectives.

The book also shows how IFS-informed EMDR is being applied in practice for PTSD and chronic pain, and with veterans, highly sensitive people, and women's group healing. In the final section, readers discover practical strategies and tools, including the Fire Drill, Jim Knipe's EMDR tools applied within IFS, and the Equid-Nexus model for equine-assisted therapy.

This comprehensive volume is ideal for anyone interested in IFS-informed EMDR and its active application by leading therapists and trainers across various contexts.

## How do you explain EMDR to your clients?

A core principle shared by both IFS and EMDR is the understanding that no one is inherently broken. The impact of trauma—or what IFS refers to as "burdens"—should not be seen as signs of pathology. Instead, these are the body's adaptive responses to perceived or real danger, developed as a need to survive.

> *The impact of trauma—or what IFS refers to as "burdens"—should not be seen as signs of pathology.*

Trauma disrupts normal memory processing, causing the body to hold unprocessed pain. Both EMDR and IFS recognize the body's capacity to heal and let go of pain.

As therapists, our job is to create a caring environment and witness the healing process. Trauma can leave people feeling powerless or disconnected. By combining IFS and EMDR, we help clients discover their inner sense of grounding, strength, and wholeness. In that space, something profound emerges—a deep knowing that they are worthy of love and care, and that their presence carries something meaningful to offer the world.

## What is your approach to addressing ambivalence or hesitation when introducing EMDR to clients?

Ambivalence is a natural and essential part of the healing process. IFS views ambivalence as multiple parts pulling in different directions. When two parts want opposing things, IFS refers to this as "polarization." Sometimes that polarization is evident in the realm of healing, especially when it involves working with burdened "exiles." This might show up as a client wondering, "Do I even want to work on my trauma?"

Some "protector" parts carry valid concerns about allowing access to exiles. At the same time, both clients and therapists may have parts that urgently want to release pain and connect with the exile. These parts may want to push past the more cautious protectors, but often, the harder they push, the more the protectors resist. Ironically, when the parts that want healing can soften and listen to the protectors they're battling, the system can find relief more quickly.

> *When the parts that want healing can soften and listen to the protectors they're battling, the system can find relief more quickly.*

Holding space for these fearful parts—and listening to what they have to say—is essential to the healing journey. When these parts feel accepted and understood, they begin to trust—and may start to loosen their grip.

When protectors refuse access to exiles, it's because they sense danger—real or perceived—and want us to understand it. Sometimes, other parts, inside the therapist or client, are impatient or frustrated with the hesitant protectors. IFS offers language for this: We can ask the urgent parts, both in ourselves and in our clients: "Would you be willing to step back just a little so we can listen directly to the part that's concerned?"

Often, these passionate parts just want acknowledgment, and when they receive it, they're willing to soften. I say, "You don't have to leave. You're welcome to stay nearby. We want to hear your message. But can we first hear what the concerned part needs us to know?" More often than not, they allow us to turn our attention toward the cautious parts—and that's when things begin to shift.

## What advice do you have for new EMDR therapists?

If you're newly trained in EMDR, I would like to begin by honoring your decision to step into this powerful and meaningful work. EMDR is a profound healing modality, and the learning curve can sometimes feel overwhelming. It's completely normal to experience self-doubt or discouragement in the early stages. If that's happening for you, know that you're not alone.

Here are a few guiding principles that have supported me on this path:

**Take your time.** In my experience, there's no substitute for the wisdom that comes from time, practice, and being in the room with clients. Let the material settle at a pace that feels right for you.

**Stay open to lifelong learning.** Ongoing consultation—and doing your own inner work—are both essential supports for growth. There's always more to discover, and that's part of what makes this work beautiful.

**Trust your inner knowing.** Trauma work brings us into sacred and vulnerable territory. Remember: To begin EMDR training, you've already completed graduate-level education and clinical training, or are on a supervised track. That means you already bring clinical judgment, relational wisdom, and ethical training to this work. These resources help you attune to your clients, listen closely to their systems, and make thoughtful decisions about when and how to proceed. You hold wisdom already—listen to it.

*You hold wisdom already—listen to it.*

## What training has had the greatest impact on your practice?

If someone is trained in EMDR but hasn't been introduced to IFS, the Syzygy Institute offers a two-day intensive workshop covering the foundational elements of Internal Family Systems. Since I had already completed IFS training, I began with Syzygy's Step 2 workshop, which provides a clear road map for integrating IFS with EMDR.

The third workshop in the series takes a deeper dive into phase 2 resourcing. Instead of relying on external imagery or strategies, it reframes resourcing as activating the client's internal adaptive information processing (AIP) network. This shift—installing internal rather than external resources—had a profound impact on how I support clients preparing for reprocessing.

To illustrate how the Syzygy model facilitates this integration, particularly for those new to it, let's look at a few core IFS concepts. Internal Family Systems is based on the idea that our psyches are made up of subpersonalities, or "parts." These parts carry stories, roles, and emotions, and often become highly activated—and can even take over our system—as a result of trauma. Healing begins when these parts are witnessed, understood, and validated—not by the therapist alone, but by what IFS calls the "Self."

The Self is our innate healing intelligence. It can also be seen as our core being, inner light, or deepest center. According to IFS, the Self cannot be damaged or lost—it is always within us. IFS describes it using eight qualities known as the "8 Cs": compassion, curiosity, clarity, calm, courage, confidence, connection, and creativity.

When clients connect with their parts and begin building relationships with them, the Self naturally begins to emerge. The Syzygy model views Self-energy as another way to understand the AIP network, the part of the system that knows how to heal.

As EMDR therapists, we help clients look inward and notice which parts are activated. In the preparation phase, we often work with protector parts—those that keep clients safe and prevent overwhelm. Before reprocessing, we ask clients not only for consent, but to check internally whether all parts feel ready to proceed. This shift, from client-level permission to system-level permission, feels more respectful and leads to deeper safety and trust.

The Syzygy model has helped me become more attuned to who I'm working with at any given moment in EMDR. *Am I engaging a protector or an exile? Is the client's Self online?* The model has given me a new lens for understanding resistance, pacing, and the relational field. Most of all, it has shown me that healing doesn't come from fixing; it comes from relationships.

> *Healing doesn't come from fixing; it comes from relationships.*

## What is one therapeutic approach that integrates really well with EMDR?

Coherence Therapy integrates beautifully with EMDR, especially when informed by Internal Family Systems. Rooted in the neuroscience of memory reconsolidation, Coherence Therapy helps us understand how even the most distressing symptoms make emotional sense when seen through the lens of lived experience.

Bruce Ecker's work on memory reconsolidation teaches that emotional learning can be transformed when we bring a previously unconscious emotional memory into awareness and pair it—repeatedly—with new information that feels deeply true but contradicts the original learning. This is more than insight; it's a neurobiological process of rewriting.

In IFS-informed EMDR, this happens when we connect with an exile and witness its pain. As the Self brings compassion, clarity, and presence, the exile is gently exposed to new information that challenges its core beliefs. When this new truth is experienced repeatedly—and paired with bilateral stimulation—the part begins to reprocess and release its old emotional learning. This is memory reconsolidation in action.

Together, these modalities offer a powerful synergy: the precision of EMDR, the relational depth of IFS, and the change mechanism of Coherence Therapy all working toward transformation from the inside out.

## What creative modifications have you made to EMDR to address specific populations or presenting issues?

When working with most clients, I find we're often addressing complex trauma. Unless someone comes in with a single-event trauma, most clients carry layers of developmental wounds and attachment injuries. For these clients, the deepest work often happens in phases 2 and 2.5 ("the Discovery Phase"), while phases 3 through 7 may be shorter or more fluid. That doesn't mean these later phases lack depth; it simply means the pace is determined by the system and sometimes unfolds more quickly once internal safety is established.

Phase 2.5 was developed by Bruce Hersey for use when protector parts are blended and the client doesn't feel safe enough to access trauma memories. These protectors often signal that there isn't enough Self-energy to proceed with standard reprocessing.

In this phase, BLS is used while engaging directly with the protector to understand its role. As trust builds, Self-energy increases and exiled parts may begin to gently emerge once the system feels safe enough.

As we move into phases 3 through 7, we continually ask: "What part am I working with right now?" In IFS-informed EMDR, we target traumatic memories held by a specific part. We use dual awareness with the part's memory only when we have (a) permission from all parts and (b) a critical mass of Self-energy online.

> *We continually ask: "What part am I working with right now?"*

In phase 3, we gather the image, negative cognition, emotion, and body sensation from the part. The part can also rate disturbance (SUD) and VOC. The client's Self offers the positive cognition.

In phase 4, we add bilateral stimulation and allow the part's pain to be noticed by the Self. The exile is seen, its injuries witnessed. The Self brings new meaning to old wounds. It offers the 8 Cs: curiosity, clarity, calm, creativity, courage, confidence, connection, and compassion. When the exile releases the burden, it is no longer defined by the trauma. We then invite it to ask the universe what qualities it would like to receive.

In phase 5, we gently reintroduce other parts to the healed exile. These parts can now form new internal relationships. Some protectors may even release their own burdens.

Throughout this process, we continue checking in with the client's body (phase 6). If intense emotions arise, we apply grounding and containment strategies that honor the client's pacing and internal safety (phase 7).

## How has your approach to EMDR evolved since you first completed your training?

When Francine Shapiro developed EMDR in the 1980s, she knew she had made a powerful discovery. At the same time, it's understandable that she may have worried it would be dismissed as radical or unsubstantiated. Would people question whether she was just another snake-oil salesperson exploiting vulnerable clients?

To gain legitimacy in the mainstream therapy world, she employed rigorous scientific methods to validate the effectiveness of EMDR. Thanks to her persistence and clarity, EMDR became an evidence-based model recognized worldwide.

I wonder if certain dynamics in the EMDR community still reflect the early struggle for legitimacy, shaped by those initial challenges. The need to protect EMDR's standing in the scientific community is both understandable and important. Still, as our understanding of trauma deepens—especially through neuroscience—it becomes essential that EMDR evolves and remains flexible.

EMDR is an incredibly helpful map for navigating the psyche, but like any model, it has limitations. What matters most is that we meet our clients with humanity and compassion—co-regulating through our nervous systems, not just techniques. Models matter, but they should be held lightly. If a model doesn't resonate with a client, we must remain open to alternatives that better meet their needs.

*What matters most is that we meet our clients with humanity and compassion—co-regulating through our nervous systems, not just techniques.*

Learning Internal Family Systems and later integrating it with EMDR was transformative for my practice. It allowed me to move with greater flexibility, attunement, and respect for the internal systems of both my clients and myself.

## What self-care practices do you engage in regularly?

Ongoing support is foundational to doing this work with integrity and sustainability. By prioritizing my own healing spaces, I've found I can show up more fully and authentically for the people I serve.

IFS-informed EMDR has deepened my understanding of my internal system and helped me recognize which parts are activated during clinical work. When I'm aware of these parts, I can turn toward them with curiosity and ask what they need. Working with my own therapist has been vital—not just for personal healing, but for my ability to accompany clients into deeper territory.

A phrase often heard in the IFS community resonates deeply: "We can only take our clients as far as we've gone with our own system."

## References

Andrew, S. R. (2023). Listening deeply. Spiritwind LLC.

Brayer, R. (2024). The art and science of EMDR: Helping clinicians bridge the path from protocol to practice. PESI Publishing.

Ecker, B., Ticic, R., & Hulley, L. (2024). Unlocking the emotional brain: Eliminating symptoms at their roots using memory reconsolidation (2nd ed.). Routledge.

Polidi, D., & McGoldrick, A. (Eds.). (2025). IFS-informed EMDR: Creative and collaborative approaches. Routledge.

Rogers, F. G., Jr. (2023). Cradled in the arms of compassion: A spiritual journey from trauma to recovery. Lake Drive Books.

# Afterword

In her book *EMDR as an Integrative Psychotherapy Approach*, Francine Shapiro makes the case that EMDR is integrative by design. It brings together the parts of a person's lived experience that shape their symptoms and suffering. I found myself returning to that framing as I worked my way through this book. EMDR is not just a set of steps you follow. It is a way of helping the nervous system metabolize what was too much, too fast, too soon, so that what is stuck can finally move.

One theme that stands out across these chapters is how often the contributors conceptualize EMDR through an attachment lens. Not everyone shares the same perspective, and not all contributors agree on this topic. But the same idea returns again and again: When the therapeutic relationship is safe enough and when repair is possible, the work goes deeper. You can hear it in how therapists pace reprocessing, how they respond to protectors, and how they stay present in the moments when a client needs the therapist more than the protocol.

You also see, again and again, how creativity is not a detour from fidelity. It is often the pathway into what words cannot reach. A symbol in a sandtray, a line of poetry, a simple image that captures a whole survival strategy, a metaphor that gives a client permission to feel without being flooded. In more than one story, it is not the retelling of trauma that creates the shift. It is the experience of being met, being welcomed, and being allowed to make meaning from what happened and what did not happen. That is whole-person work, and it is part of why EMDR is so much more than a set of protocols.

I am deeply grateful to every contributor in this book. Their generosity is obvious on the page, and it also reflects how they live: being there for clients, for consultees, and for each other. If this book leaves you feeling more inspired, that is because the contributors were willing to share what they have learned with honesty, with humility, and with heart.

If you want community as you continue to grow, I hope you will join The EMDR Learning Community (emdr-learning.com). It is free, and it exists for one reason: so you do not have to do this work alone. In a world that can feel fragmented and harsh, choosing healing is a form of unity, and I invite you to be part of it.

www.ingramcontent.com/pod-product-compliance
Lightning Source LLC
LaVergne TN
LVHW100322210926
848480LV00003B/1215
*9798994806005*